Workable Sisterhood

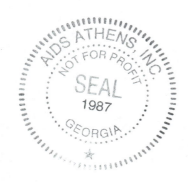

Workable Sisterhood

THE POLITICAL JOURNEY OF
STIGMATIZED WOMEN WITH HIV/AIDS

Michele Tracy Berger

PRINCETON UNIVERSITY PRESS
PRINCETON AND OXFORD

Second printing, and first paperback printing, 2006
Paperback ISBN-13: 978-0-691-12770-5
Paperback ISBN-10: 0-691-12770-0

The Library of Congress has cataloged the cloth edition
of this book as follows

Berger, Michele Tracy, 1968–
Workable sisterhood : the political journey of stigmatized
women with HIV/AIDS /
Michele Tracy Berger.
p.   cm.
Includes bibliographical references and index.
ISBN 0-691-11853-1 (cl : alk. paper)
1. Women with social disabilities—United States—Political activity.
2. HIV-positive women—United States—Political activity.   3. Political participation—
United States.   4. Marginality, Social—United States.   5. AIDS (Disease)—Social
aspects—United States.   6. Stigma (Social psychology)
I. Title.

HQ1236.5.U6B495 2004
362.83'0973—dc22   2003066414

British Library Cataloging-in-Publication Data is available

This book has been composed in Janson

Printed on acid-free paper. ∞

pup.princeton.edu

Printed in the United States of America

10 9 8 7 6 5 4 3 2

*For the many unnamed brave women living
in the United States with the HIV/AIDS virus*

Contents

Acknowledgments

I would like to thank the pioneering spirit of scholars Cathy Cohen, Nancy Stoller, and Lisa Maher. Their research has been a source of great inspiration.

I am grateful for early believers in my work including: Martha Feldman, Kathleen Daly, Janet Hart, Mary Corcoran, Kim Lane Scheppele, Beth Glover, Catherine West-Newman, and Carol Boyd. Gratitude also goes to Jonah Levy, Judy Gruber, Donald Rosenthal, and Ted Jelen, who provided excellent suggestions during various stages of this project. Thanks also go to Irene Rosenfeld for her shrewd and discerning editorial assistance.

I would like to thank the generous support of the Robert Wood Johnson Foundation's Health Policy Research Scholars Program. I am also appreciative of the support I received while a participant in the Scholars Program from the University of California, Berkeley, School of Public Health which provided the space, resources, and intellectual camaraderie necessary to conclude this book.

An author could not ask for a more receptive editor than Chuck Myers. Through every stage of the process he allayed fears, provided clear instructions and enthusiastic feedback. Ellen Foos's direction and guidance as production editor was invaluable. Additional thanks goes to Jennifer Nippins for her assistance stewarding the manuscript through the many administrative routes that lead to publication.

For the unflagging support and affirmation from the following, I wish to thank Kathleen Guidroz, Jodi O'Brien, Jodi Sandfort, Steve Marchese, Ajuan Mance, Cassandra Falby, and Barbara Wallace. Lastly, I'd like to thank Timothy Dane Keim for his excellent companionship, encouragement, and impeccable nature.

Workable Sisterhood

## CHAPTER ONE

The Politics of Intersectional Stigma for Women with HIV/AIDS

I am sitting in a living room, in Detroit, full of decoratively placed plants. The colorful plants help to make the sparsely furnished room feel comfortable. My attention is drawn back to Nicole,[1] a forty-two-year-old African American woman sitting in front of me on the couch. She is wearing an amber colored dress. Her braids are held back by an attractive hair tie, and she possesses a clear cadence to her voice. We have been talking for about an hour, and all my senses are alert. Nicole is about to tell me more of her recent political projects. From a manila folder, Nicole pulls out some materials to show me. Her file is crammed with press clippings, letters from Congresspeople, and grant applications.

Nicole is a former sex worker,[2] former small-time drug dealer, and former crack addict. She contracted HIV[3] five years ago; she has been and continues to be a stigmatized woman. Yet these categories alone I mention above contribute little to understanding her life when she was those other things, nor, more importantly, what her life has become now. She is a woman living with HIV who has become politically engaged. She is one of the foremost people involved with women and AIDS activism in Detroit. That afternoon we talk about Detroit politics, black male and female relationships, and prostitution. After talking with Nicole I feel that I am on to "something" about women and political engagement; I am learning from her. (Fieldnote 1996)

THIS FIELDNOTE, written in 1996, initiated a new way of thinking about the various women I had been studying in Detroit. What had begun several years ago as a research inquiry into the status of female lawbreakers,[4] a "story" about crime, prostitution, and the ravages of crack cocaine use, had instead over time become transformed into a "story" explicating the lives of stigmatized, politically active HIV-positive women.[5] This story was recast to highlight women (formerly active female lawbreakers) who after being diagnosed with the HIV/AIDS virus changed their lives. Finally, it evolved into a story about stigma, struggle, and a group of women who are nontraditional political actors. The process of how Nicole and other women reconstituted their lives once they became HIV-positive, how they created and utilized a web of nontraditional resources and participated in their communities became the cornerstone of this research. Their life struggles and political involvement help to question what scholars know about political participation for stigmatized women. The process by which these women have transformed themselves and exerted their rights in a democratic society deserves scholarly attention— and is a story worth telling.

There are three central elements to this story, making this story worthy of further explication. They are the actors (the women), the event (acquiring the HIV/AIDS virus), and the outcome (their political participation). Each of the elements is interdependent with the others, and they work together to create meaning. The questions that emerge from the telling of this story include: (1) How does such a severely stigmatized group of women participate? (2) Why do they participate? (3) What types of activities constitute participation for the women?

This chapter provides an overview of how the women "arrived" at this moment as politicized people, and what this arrival epistemologically ushers forth for capturing the dimensions of stigma and participation. Throughout, I reframe central questions about what constitutes political participation, including: How can we expand the notion of politics to include my respondents' experiences? Drawing on sociological insights about "community work" as political, I argue that in order to capture the dimensions of stigmatized women's work in their communities, a much more generous assessment of politics must be deployed. In the second half, I introduce the theoretical framework of intersectional stigma that helps explain the challenges stigmatized people face when becoming politically active. Intersectional stigma furthers the investigation into how people are situated within axes of social identities that often confer power and privilege.

Let us now return to the respondents. We begin with an overview of the story, followed by an argument designed to broaden our notions of politics.

AN OVERVIEW OF THE STORY

Sixteen women's lives comprise the foundation of this study. Their life stories are neither transparent nor easy for a researcher to characterize. Before becoming HIV-positive, most had lived lives that would make them suspect to the majority of Americans. They are primarily women of color.[6] They were sex workers, drug users (primarily of crack cocaine), and lawbreakers (engaging in criminalized activities) in every sense of the word. Personally, many of these women's lives were complicated by domestic violence, childhood sexual trauma, sexual assault, family substance use, and intermittent poverty. Before they became HIV-positive, aspects of their lives could be characterized as troubled, difficult, unmanageable, and depressing. They were women whom the average person would not have taken notice of, identified with, nor thought worthy of any special attention. If anything, they were women whom society had either given up on or directed particular punitive policies, agendas, and programs against.[7]

These sixteen women were diagnosed with the HIV/AIDS virus from 1986 to 1996. During their diagnosis, they were perceived and identified by medical providers and others involved in the medical arena already as "deviant" women. The circumstances surrounding how the women discovered their HIV-positive condition might surprise, or even shock, the average person. The experiences they recounted were humiliating, painful, and stigmatizing. I have labeled their remembrances, and subsequent actions because of these remembrances, under the rubric *narratives of injustice*. The narratives of injustice suggest to us the mistreatment the women faced due to the specific conditions of their experience. These events created the catalyst for respondents to embark upon an individual and collective quest grappling with what it meants to be a stigmatized HIV-positive woman.

Collectively, these women represent populations (women of color, drug users, urban residents, low-income women, drug-using prostitutes) that are among the fastest growing groups in the country with HIV/AIDS. They represent the new "face" of populations with HIV/AIDS in this country. They are a group of women with HIV who are highly stigmatized because of their former lifestyles. Also, because they have overlapping membership within the groups mentioned, they embody the structural ways in which the disease highlights long-standing areas of inequality along race, class, and gender axes.

Infection with the HIV/AIDS virus has the capacity to make previously *hidden* people public. Groups who were marginalized before (e.g., gay male communities) have come into public view because of the ravages of HIV/AIDS. For some, however, this disease can increase invisibility, causing individuals to recede further into marginality and stigmatization. Some people respond to the public labeling of HIV, and resulting stigma, with resignation, shame, and death. This story, about these women, could have ended here without another passing thought. But it does not.

There are other HIV-positive people who refuse to be made invisible, who use their rage and fear to mobilize and confront existing power structures. The women discussed here fall into this category. The rest of the story is about how these sixteen women responded to the HIV/AIDS crisis in personal ways that spiraled out to touch and intersect with their communities and the political realm.

Intersectional stigma is a distinctive aspect of their story. What makes their experience of the HIV/AIDS virus and their participation different from other counterparts of people with HIV is the influence of intersectional stigma. Intersectional stigma is a theoretical framework composed of the recognition of and attention to *intersectionality* (or acknowledgment of race, class, and gender subordination as interlocking forms of oppression), and *stigma* (or the ways in which people become socially defined as "other"). Intersectional stigma allows me to theorize about the distinct ways in which marginality is manifested and experienced. Furthermore, intersectional stigma represents the total synchronistic influence of various forms of oppression, which combine and overlap to form a distinct *positionality*.

Through the prism of intersectional stigma, we can theorize that given that the women were *already* socially positioned as "deviant women," the effect of the HIV/AIDS virus was to dramatically add to and combine with their existing social marginality. This phenomenon, I argue, is in part related to the fact that contracting the HIV/AIDS virus as a woman who has a crack cocaine and sex work background is incredibly stigmatizing. The framework of intersectional stigma helps explain the reasons why when initially diagnosed with HIV they received negative treatment from family, medical providers, peers, and others. Because of the onus of intersectional stigma, they experienced a qualitatively distinct form of stigma. Additionally, their HIV-positive status and experience of intersectional stigma highlighted other facets of inequality in their lives. Coming to terms with *why* they were stigmatized as people with HIV forced them to ask deeper questions of themselves. The questions once raised would cause a search for answers, which would continue to change and shape their lives.

Through this process they embarked on the path of "life reconstruction." Life reconstruction is the underlying foundation facilitating women's political activities; it consists of the specific ways in which women redirected areas of stigma that enabled them to deal with the HIV/AIDS virus. The result of this process was minimally twofold. First, it enabled them to develop a "public voice" about being a woman with HIV; second, it allowed them to become aware of resources that would form the underpinning for their later political activities. The resources gained by the women during the life reconstruction process were not usually those of professional status and mobility, higher education, or large amounts of money. These are the resources usually associated with political participation. The women, however, discovered and developed both external and internal resources including faith and spirituality, substance abuse treatment, therapeutic work on early sexual trauma, a reliance on self and female peers, an introduction to HIV/AIDS advocacy, and ideas about activism.

Regarding political participation, there is a generally accepted idea of a hierarchy of mobilization. This idea suggests that a person often begins being politically active at the "lower" end of the spectrum, and then moves into the "higher" end. Or, stated another way, a person moves from informal to formal political activity. Political activity is often not seen as an end within itself, but a constant progressing toward more complex forms of participation (Rosenstone and Hansen 1993; Ackelsberg 1988). Interviews with the politically active HIV-positive women forced me to reexamine this theoretical "hierarchy of mobilization" from these women's perspectives.

For my respondents, participation did not emerge as the result of an isolated, abstract process, a process that is so often described by many political participation scholars; their participation is embedded in a relational dynamic (for critiques of the democratic process as isolated, abstract, and universally male see Ackelsberg 1988; Bookman and Morgen 1988; Flammang 1997; Nelson 1989).

When we think of people exerting political power and influence in our society, we tend to think of people casting votes, forming political action committees, or deciding to run for office. Yet many types of political "work" hold American society together. With a renewed sense of optimism, and faith, the women, through their efforts, slowly became part of the political process and affected the lives of HIV-positive people. And yet their participation did not culminate with someone running for office—providing for an easy, neat, and linear ending to their participation and the story.

The best method to capture the ways in which they articulated the work they did in their communities and the meanings they made from it is reflected in my concept of *blended and overlapping roles*. Blended and overlapping roles draw on the structure of their paid and unpaid activities in the community. Their use of blended and overlapping roles also allowed them to draw on various kinds of knowledge and expertise.

The Women and the Activities

The activities respondents participate in range from "formal" political action like voting to "informal" political action. Most respondents have moved into various types of grass-roots-level political participation, primarily in the areas of HIV/AIDS issues. These latter activities include undertaking HIV/AIDS outreach and education; petitioning the state of Michigan for monies for HIV/AIDS research conducted on women; and fighting for better substance abuse treatment programs for lower-income women. They have petitioned the legislature about bills that would affect HIV-positive people. Other participants have attended national conferences (as panelists and invited presenters) and have spoken to women and young girls at different facilities including prisons, churches, schools, and community centers. A few have made appearances on both radio and television; others have written opinion pieces for newspapers. Women's efforts have resulted in the widespread usage of pre- and posttreatment counselors in most HIV/AIDS testing sites. Working with city officials, they have advocated for better-designed support and service programs for women with HIV and their children. Some have helped design those programs. They have testified in public hearings related to HIV/AIDS issues. Many of these activities helped them to stay both self-empowered and community focused.

Broadly construed, the primary concerns of my respondents that lead to political engagement include HIV/AIDS education, HIV/AIDS prevention, health care, child welfare, community development, and crime. Overall, these types of informal and grass-roots-level organizing are thought of as a common pathway for women as first political experiences (Randall 1987; West and Blumberg 1990).

To continue this discussion it is appropriate to look closely at the situation of U.S. women with the HIV/AIDS virus. Just what has been the virus's impact on women in the last decade?

THE NEW "FACE" OF HIV/AIDS

> *The women HIV affects are more varied than the virus's own mutations.*
>
> *Nothing better epitomizes the multiple voices and visions of AIDS than women's experiences of the epidemic.*
>
> —Nancy Stoller, *Lessons from the Damned*

The HIV/AIDS virus is a pandemic issue. The United States is undergoing a significant shift in the populations the virus is affecting. Women continue to increase as AIDS patients (Phillips 1997).[8] Deaths caused by AIDS declined in men during 1996, but increased in women by 3 percent (Phillips 1997). This change has come in what seems like a short span of time, little more than a decade. The HIV/AIDS virus is now seen as reaching a plateau for some groups of men in the United States, but still swelling for women. The acquisition and treatment of HIV/AIDS in this country underscores several of the structural realities of class, race, and gender. Among women of color, African American women, in particular, have been hard hit by the spread of the virus:

Between 1985 and 1988, the rate of HIV-infection quadrupled among women of color, many of whom reside in poverty-stricken inner city communities. Today, women of color constitute 72% of all women infected with HIV, 53% of whom are African American and 20% of whom are from Latin America. Urban mortality rates indicate that AIDS is the leading cause of death among African American women between the ages of 15 and 44 years and among Latinas between the ages of 25 and 34 in New York and New Jersey. It is predicted that in the twenty-first century, AIDS will become the leading crusade of death among minority women of childbearing age. (Chu, Buschler, and Berkelman 1990; as cited in Land 1994, 356)

By recent Center for Disease Control and Prevention (CDC) statistics AIDS is *now* the third leading cause of death for African American women among the age group of twenty-five to forty-four. AIDS among African American women could be considered a crisis that affects not only individual women but their communities (see Land 1994). HIV/AIDS risks for black women, as for other women, are complicated by structural factors of inequality.

Women acquire the HIV/AIDS virus from different routes of transmission than men. Drug use, particularly intravenous drug use, as well as an exacerbating influence of sex-for-crack exchanges have been implicated as contributing to the rise of infection among women (Phillips 1997). Although drug use was known in the early days as a factor contributing to HIV/AIDS transmission, recent information has shown that it is of greater importance than previously believed. Additionally, the co-determining phenomenon of various types of drug use, the prevalence of certain drugs in large urban areas, and the fact that the majority of women infected live in cities with populations over 500,000 all speak to the interrelated problems of race, class, gender, and marginality (Phillips 1997). It is now an agreed-upon observation that Stoller acknowledges: "HIV among women is a disease of the poor, uneducated, and the ghettoized" (1998, 11). The degree to which women have been affected by the disease is inseparable from the historical scars of inequality in American society.

WOMEN'S COMMUNITY WORK: BROADENING THE DEFINITION OF WHAT CONSTITUTES POLITICS

In the last twenty-five years there have been a number of revisions to the traditional understanding of women and politics, moving away from gender as a simple and transparent category to a growing interest in gender as a multifaceted dimension of analysis. This has produced central questions, arguments, and revisions of what constitutes the political terrain for women. Janet Flammang succinctly discusses the ways in which dominant approaches in understanding women's political participation are lacking:

In order to understand women's political participation, conceptual lenses needed to be refocused in three ways: from the military state to the social welfare state, from the state to the community, and from interest groups to voluntary associations. (1997, 96)

Flammang's insight is precisely astute for this discussion. The new theoretical investigations for gender and political participation involve redefining what activities constitute the "political," particularly as it intersects with what has been called "community work." Community work encompasses a diverse array of activities that fall in the realm of nonelectoral participation.

Until recently, examination of working-class women's and lower-income women's political activities in their communities had been missing from the rubric of women, politics, and participation (Bookman and Morgen 1988). Bookman and Morgen (1988) helped spark this new direction by arguing for an overall redefinition of politics to include activities women are routinely immersed in. These activities include grass-roots-level organizing in the communities in which they live. Moreover, investigations into activities that define "community work" and the terrain of women's links in communities have begun to counter that absence. This new direction is helpful in countering the assumption that certain types of women *do not* politically participate. There have been significant reconceptualizations of politics through multidisciplinary inquiry, which combine questions of women's political agency, community activism, and race, class, and gender analyses (see Naples 1998). The scholarship originates from diverse sources, including multiethnic studies, history, anthropology, and sociology. Activists and community organizers have also contributed to this literature. Recent interest in community work has also been fueled by interest in how the "war on poverty" programs created state-funded employment and volunteer positions that women primarily filled (see Gilkes 1988, 1994; Naples 1991a).

As women's activism at the community level is being unearthed, it portrays a historically and theoretically different picture of women's politicization from what we have come to believe. Traditional categories used to ascertain women's participation have masked women's militancy (Naples 1991b). Additionally, the idea that all participation comes from general self-interest is a model that does not resonate with women's forms of participation and reasons for participation (Ackelsberg 1988). Women's involvement in charitable organizations to community groups has been an important part of women's political landscape (Cott 1987; Giddings 1984). Naples argues the study of women's community-based activism in the twentieth century "has also contributed significantly to the re-conceptualization of sociological categories—especially 'politics,' 'work,' and 'family' typically used to analyze social life" (1998, 3). Naples asserts that "women's unpaid work and community activism were essential for the formation of the modern social welfare state" (1991a, 318).

It is precisely the ways in which scholars are conceptualizing community level organizing (also referred to as "community work") and other forms of participation that begin to illuminate the activities of the Detroit women. Much of the work they engage in is on behalf of the HIV-positive community and includes informal participation. Our current ideas about participation have to be broadened to include community work that involves paid and unpaid labor.

Some scholars have investigated how women's community unpaid and paid work is connected with and intersects the political realm (Naples 1994; Gilkes 1980, 1988). Scholars have argued that community work and notions of community highlight avenues of social change: "One of the most consistent themes to emerge from feminist analyses of women's political praxis is the significance of constructions of community for women's politicization and social action" (Naples 1998, 330).

Community work has been defined two different ways in the sociological inquiry into women's activities: as paid and unpaid activities. Community work has often been defined as work or labor outside the home: "It is the labor these women perform often in addition to work in the household and the labor force" (Gilkes 1994, 230). Community work can constitute nonelectoral forms of participation that serve to help, define, and protect a community against external threats. Some studies of community work highlight the ways in which women of color have worked to mitigate racism in their communities (see Gilkes 1988; Naples 1994).

Gilkes has written extensively on the role of community activism by middle-class African American women (see 1980, 1983, 1988, 1990, 1994). She studies how a number of African American women working for the state (programs developed in response to antipoverty campaigns) helped create a voice for the ongoing struggles of racism directed at their communities; they often served as an interface between state and local agencies.[9] She details how some black women constructed professional careers through the avenues of community work while simultaneously fighting on behalf of community interest. Gilkes (1994) argues that this type of sustained effort can be a route community workers utilize to synchronistically challenge racism. Community work, Gilkes documents, itself covers a "wide range of tasks":

> Community work consists of the women's activities to combat racism and empower their communities to survive, grow, and advance in a hostile society. The totality of their work is an emergent, dynamic, interactive model of social action in which community workers discover and explore oppressive structures, challenge many different structures and practices which keep their communities powerless and disadvantaged, and then build, maintain, and strengthen institutions within their community. These institutions become the basis for the community's political culture. The women generate an alternative organization, and a set of commitments to group interest are the basic elements of the community. They work for the community that they themselves re-create and sustain, a mutually reinforcing process. (230)

Gilkes continues to map out an expansive definition about the nature and scope of these activities. The activities she chronicles help shift the focus from macrolevel settings to microlevel settings:

> Community work is focused on internal development and external challenge, and creates ideas enabling people to think about change. It is the work that opens doors to elected and appointed positions in the political power struggle, and demands and creates jobs in local labor markets and the larger economic system. Community work also focuses on changing ideas, stereotypes, and images that keep a group perpetually *stigmatized*. . . . Community work is a constant struggle, and it consists of everything that people do to address oppression in their own lives, suffering in the lives of others and their sense of solidarity or group kinships. (231, emphasis added)

Naples has expanded on these microlevel dimensions, delving into the community work of black and Latina women whose self-defined categories did not fit with traditional conceptualizations of politics (1991a, 1991b, 1994). Naples articulates a compelling understanding of how some black women's and Latina women's activism translates into "activist mothering," where a concern for women's work in low-income neighborhoods consisted of the interconnections between political activism, mothering, community work, and paid labor (Naples 1994).[10] Her analysis of "activist mothering" captures radical notions about the political activities and "self perceptions of their motherwork" (Naples 1994). Generated from oral narratives, it challenges the traditional definitions of labor, socially reproductive work, and politics. Throughout these works there is a focus on social change and everyday politics.

One of the keys to understanding women's community work is that women maintain social affiliations and networks from communities they grew up in. These networks are drawn on for political work. Women community activists are also "politicized through specific experiences or struggles that they must first reflect upon before they can take effective action" (Naples 1998, 332). This process involves discussing feelings and ideas with others who may have had similar troubles:

> This interaction between the everyday life experiences of injustice, inequality, and abuse and processes of reflection occurring within social networks with specific gender, race, and class divisions opens spaces for oppositional consciousness and activism. The broader cultural, political, and economic environment also forms a powerful material context framing their lives and profoundly shapes how activists defined their relationship to specific struggles, what political actions might be effective, and what resources are available. It also structures the very grounds upon which many of their experiences are built. (Naples 1998, 332–33)

Race, class, and gender have not been mutually exclusive topics within studies of community work, but have been used as different kinds of conceptual focuses since the initial investigation on women's activities (see Bookman and Morgen 1988). As research emerged, women of color were documented as playing a central role in the extent to which they were participants. Probing the differences between white women and women of color community workers has been an important theoretical goal in the evolution of research on community work. Naples notes:

> However, while white women and women of color may describe their motivation for community work as an extension of their gender identities, their differing standpoints shaped by race-ethnicity, class, sexual orientation and region of residence influence how they define their family's and community's needs, as well as the political strategies to accomplish differing goals. (Naples 1992, 443; Naples 1998; Gilkes 1988; Susser 1988)

Therefore from these insights Naples challenges scholars to look to broader evidences of political activity, and argues that if "we turn our attention to the community-based work of African American, Latinas, and other women of color, we are forced to reconceptualize our understanding of community work, political activism, mothering, and by extension, our analyses of labor" (1994, 224). This expansive rubric of community work is theoretically adopted in understanding respondents' activities. As later chapters will demonstrate, this study of respondents' activities in the area of HIV/AIDS is an extension of theoretically disentangling the various layers of where and how stigmatized low-income women's participation manifests.

I argue that through their efforts they helped to create and re-create a sense of community, and that their labor overlaps and often resists easy public or private distinctions. They struggled on behalf of an extensively defined HIV-positive community. Although the focus in much of the research conducted by Gilkes (1994) and others (Sotelo-Hondagneu 1998; Pardo 1998; Park 1998; Stern 1998) has examined community work derived from definitions of community that include race, language, ethnic background, and discrimination, other research has demonstrated how women engage in community work in a wide array of settings, against a number of oppressive situations (see Bookman and Morgen 1988; Krauss 1998 for toxic waste and struggles by white working-class women; Naples 1998; Taylor and Rupp 1998 on lesbian activism; Wittner 1998 on battered women's activism). Respondents' activities fit within and expand on current research and definitions of community work. Including women's unpaid and paid activities within the HIV/AIDS arena demonstrates the broadness and flexibility of community work as a way to analyze participation on various social issues.

Moreover, incorporating insights about community work into questions about gender and political participation yields gains for both sets of inquiries. Looking at stigmatized women expands the research on community work because there has been little research that discusses the community work of severely stigmatized women. Incorporating community work within traditional inquiries of gender and political participation is a logical extension of critiques already put forth by scholars working in diverse fields. Community work captures a more comprehensive spectrum of American women, and it potentially provides an in-depth mapping of informal political participation.

We turn now to a brief explication of how roles help us to understand the Detroit women's activism and its connection to community work.

Roles

How do women work on behalf of the HIV-positive community?[11] What activities do they undertake? This question is best answered with an attention to blended and overlapping roles, roles that combine paid and unpaid work for the Detroit women. *Advocates*, *activists*, and *helpers* are the categories used to describe and explain their roles and contour of their activities. Chapter 7 documents the fluidity between the roles. These positions are self-defined and form a web of relationships with local, city, and state government. They are not solely identity based.[12] The type of activities the women engage in help define their community and are consistent with other goals that research on community work has explored. Their activities on behalf of the HIV-positive community include:

- defining the HIV-positive community
- renegotiating and redefining stigma about people and the disease, dispelling an "us versus them" mentality
- performing "face-to-face" work[13]
- creating cultural products and events about HIV
- involving themselves in the survival and quality of life of HIV-positive people
- working for material and social change

For their efforts, they have received what other scholars have called a *"community mandate"* (Gilkes 1994). The term refers to the ways in which community workers receive status or recognition from other community members for working on behalf of the community.

The role of advocate usually involves some paid work within a city agency, nonprofit organization or community center. Advocates use their positions to advance critiques of the system; Activists are women who engage in more direct confrontational strategies; they are also women who have felt somewhat marginalized in larger HIV/AIDS community projects. They are interested in producing cultural products, products that challenge negative images of HIV-positive people. Helpers are bridge women, often trained in some form of advocacy; they also facilitate other women's participation in community activities.

Not only is important for us to perceive women as political actors, but it is essential for scholars to pay attention to what venues women are politically in. As Vicky Randall suggests, interested scholars need to take note of the various activities that women engage in, activities that look less like conventional politics. These include makeshift organizations, self-help projects, popular protests, and the like. She argues that all of these arenas might be a fruitful place to look for women's sustained activity (Randall 1987). My work suggests that researchers need a reevaluation and reconceptualization both of how stigmatized women choose to organize and of where they organize or participate. Often the "sites" where they undertake political work—that is, drug treatment centers, support groups, community groups, and so forth—tend not to be recognized by researchers. For respondents, the places where political activities/community work occur straddle conventional public and private realms. The physical locations include micro- and macrolevels. Some of the macrolevel physical spaces include hospitals, churches, neighborhoods, community centers, agencies, schools, and prisons. Examples of the microlevel physical spaces include a woman's home, picnics, hair salons, support groups, and conferences (not city funded).

Features of their political process, based on their role structure, could also be categorized as experientially focused, often black-female led and participatory/community oriented.

Politics, Women, and HIV/AIDS

Scholars have begun to take interest in how HIV-positive women have become politically active and empowered.[14] The scope of this literature has evolved through the fields of public health, social work, community organizing, nursing, sociology, and anthropology. Theoretically, there has been sustained attention to how women with the HIV/AIDS virus (and others) are involved in a broadly defined HIV/AIDS social movement.

There exist methodological and theoretical gaps in terms of explaining and providing rigorous examples of the various *processes* of empowerment for women with HIV (including catalysts for participation and different routes to and expressions of participation). Early work sought to document grass-roots level organizing in various communities (ACT UP/NY Women and AIDS Book Group 1992). Most of the documentation came from activists, who were interested in making women with HIV/AIDS visible and also providing political strategizing and organizing tips for women with HIV (see Carlomusto 1992; Dixon 1992; Wolfe 1992). This work nationally documented videos, demonstrations, outreach, and peer education programs. Early on there was a recognition that social context influenced pathways to different women's HIV/AIDS participation (Schneider and Stoller 1995). For example, the homophobia as well as the medical profession's established responses that "lesbians are not at risk" worked initially to silence lesbians. Lesbian and bisexual women were involved in HIV/AIDS activism on behalf of their friends and associates in gay male communities. It was only after numerous vituperative discussions and dilemmas about what defined "lesbian sex" (and the fact that lesbian-identified women were contracting HIV) that lesbians mobilized on behalf of themselves and their community.[15]

Heterosexual women initially confronted few services tailored to women, difficulty in accesing services, and invisibility issues (i.e., "nice girls don't get HIV/AIDS"; see Grove, Kelly, and Liu 1997). They also had to face and negotiate condom use and to challenge certain types of sexual behaviors with male partners—a difficult situation for most women, given gender socialization (Schneider and Stoller 1995; Act/UP New York Women and AIDS Book Group 1992). Researchers have focused on the inadequacy of services women with HIV/AIDS face and the lack of information provided to women (see Land 1994), but the experience of being treated poorly at the time of diagnosis or the impact of multiple stigmas have not been widely discussed.

For respondents, pathways to participation and empowerment begin with the acquisition of the virus. Activity did not begin for these women until after they were diagnosed. This makes them similar to some other groups, particularly women, who found themselves HIV-positive. HIV provided a catalyst for them, but it is argued here that this was also related to the social context surrounding the acquisition of and disclosure of the virus. Their route to activism was marked with the trials and tribulations of being a stigmatized person because of drug use and prostitution. This had consequences for the information they received and how they perceived their treatment. As is discussed fully in chapter 4, the women who discovered they were HIV-positive cite the many distressing circumstances surrounding their diagnosis of the HIV/AIDS virus. Briefly, health officials did not give them proper information, and they were also given the message that the medical establishment could do nothing for them. Their impetus to change was not just the result of the HIV/AIDS virus, but it was also because they felt they were treated poorly and discriminated against (because of their drug use status and their sex work background); they felt as if they were given bad information when initially diagnosed with HIV. Misinformation with HIV/AIDS is not uncommon, as other research has suggested:

> Women of color receive greater misinformation about HIV/AIDS and underestimate personal risk (Kalichman et al. 1992; Marin 1989). Thus, they constitute a growing and vulnerable group at risk for the physical manifestations of AIDS and its psychological sequlae. (as cited in Land 1994, 356)

It has been much later that scholars have turned to the subject of HIV/AIDS and examined the specific types of leadership women have held in that arena (Schneider and Stoller 1995). Slowly, narratives about the varied experiences of women have been incorporated in the "official record," and what Stoller (1998) has called "histories of women with HIV/AIDS" have become more visible. Women on the front lines of HIV/AIDS activism as well as scholars have begun to write about the diversity of this phenomena (see Alexander 1995; Denison 1995; Fraser and Jones 1995; Greenblat 1995; Hollibaugh 1995; Lewis 1995; Lockett 1995; Stoller 1995).[16] Methodologically, these are often short reflection pieces, which try to provide an account of the complicated dynamics women with HIV have faced and responded to in the last decade (see Schneider and Stoller 1995). Schneider and Stoller (1995) outline main themes in evaluating women's leadership within the HIV/AIDS crisis:

> (1) recognizing HIV/AIDS is a pandemic issue; (2) sustained attention to the social relationship to race, class, sexuality, and culture. The third theme is feminist social change, very broadly defined from the individual to collective; (4) emphasis on women's skills and activities. (3–6)

Women who acquire the HIV/AIDS virus have used various means to increase their visibility, which include activities like developing support groups, outreach programs (set up in places from hair salons to churches), and protest demonstrations. Women who are not HIV-positive have also helped to spearhead some of these efforts, as well as been caregivers and resource people. Schneider and Stoller note the possibility for potential social change:

> Consequently, women are in strategic positions to affect the course of HIV's spread. Because of gender segregation in the workplace, women are the vast majority of employees in caregiving and health professions and seem to be the majority of workers in AIDS service organizations in most locations in the world. (1995, 1)

The political work women have undertaken has been constructed to help a larger populace who have direct stakes with women and HIV/AIDS issues, including policy makers, sex educators, social workers, health personnel, and the like (Schneider and Stoller 1995).

Throughout these analyses, the same problems emerge for understanding stigmatized women—it turns on the question of Who gets studied? As Schneider and Stoller acknowledge, early work on HIV/AIDS activism did not focus on outsider groups:

> Poor women are often portrayed as unskilled, passive, and uninterested in politics. Like other struggles of poor and working-class women, the political worlds affected by the epidemic have been obscured and the activities of white, middle-class women have received most of the attention. In the AIDS epidemic, poor, working class and middle-class women are all actively engaged in efforts to change their lives and the institutions that serve them. (1995, 5)

This literature, while useful in its focus on women's politicizing activities and HIV/AIDS, is conceptually lacking in its ability to help further explain the process of political consciousness that defines the group of women studied. As noted earlier, the pathways to participation are different for this group of women with HIV; so too is their process of political consciousness. The process(es) for women with HIV in relation to self-empowerment and political activity have not been sufficiently teased out by scholars.

Focusing on process allows for the dynamism of the women's experiences in the sample to come to light. The phrase "life reconstruction" is used to signify the specific identifiable processes that allow women to construct, expand, reshape, or begin anew what it means to be a *woman with HIV*. The life reconstruction process also brought them into contact with specific resources, resources not usualy identified by researchers.

There are two major components that define the life reconstruction process. They are substance use treatment/recovery and gender identity. Substance abuse treatment plays a central role in the beginning of the process; substance abuse treatment often provides a stable and supportive place for the women.

Schneider and Stoller (1995) suggest that women with the HIV/AIDS virus have to recast themselves and their roles within the private sphere. This focus on gender and political consciousness for respondents in my study is to capture the "micro-processes of gender socialization" (Schneider and Stoller 1995). This is especially fruitful inquiry, given that many of these women had previously either negative experiences with being a woman or had focused on other central features of their identity. One of the more tangible outcomes of this life reconstruction process for the women is the development of a "public voice."

In summary, although there is a recognition of the importance of stigma (see Act/UP Women and AIDS Book Group 1992), there is scant research about how the pathways, context, and process of empowerment might differ for different social groups of women. When discussing the role of activism, concepts related to advocacy as gained through substance abuse treatment are rarely mentioned. There is also not recognition that some women may overlap their HIV/AIDS advocacy with other roles or advocacy positions in their community. All of these factors are important considerations in capturing the picture of HIV-positive women's community involvement.

Politics of Everyday Life

Embedded in the midst of this discussion of community work is the question of what defines political activity. Some scholars have argued that traditional versions of politics do little to explain how marginalized people experience the world (Cohen 1993; Kelley 1994). What community work often captures is the process of how people deal with "the politics of everyday life." This dynamic interplay is quite hard to capture statistically or even to conceptualize outside formal political activity.

In this study, there are three sets of ideas about politics that are drawn on in assessing, explaining, and evaluating the activities of respondents. One focus is on empowerment, a term often mentioned by respondents in helping themselves and people in their communities. Bookman and Morgen use this definition in their work as a central concept in reframing politics for women:

> empowerment begins when they [women] change their ideas about the causes of their powerlessness, when they recognize the systemic forces that oppress them, and when they act to change the conditions of their lives. (1988, 4)

Naples in her study of women community workers offers her conceptualization, or schema, of "doing politics":

> doing politics included any struggle to gain control over definitions of "self" and "community"; to augment personal and communal empowerment; to create alternative institutions and organizational processes; and to increase the power and resources of their community. (1991b, 479)

Finally, Robin Kelley, a historian, argues in his study of black working-class politics and culture that one must look at the margins, and go beyond what we think we know about politics to investigate new forms and meanings (1994). He suggests that sometimes "dynamic struggles take place—outside—indeed, sometimes in spite of—established organizations and institutions" (7). Kelley urges scholars to pay attention to the reasons why people participate, as opposed to solely studying the outcomes of participation:

> Too often politics is defined by *how* people participate rather than *why*; by traditional definition the question of what is political hinges on whether or not groups are involved in elections, political parties, or grass-roots social movements. Yet, the how seems far less important than the why, since many of the so-called real

political institutions have not always proved effective for, or even accessible to, oppressed people. . . . I am rejecting the tendency to dichotomize people's lives, to assume that clear-cut "political" motivations exist separately from issues of economic well-being, safety, pleasure, cultural expression, sexuality, freedom of mobility, and other facets of daily life. Politics is not separate from lived experience or the imaginary world of what is possible; to the contrary, politics is about these things, as to roll back constraints and exercise some power over, or create some space within, the institutions and social relationships that dominate our lives. (10, emphasis in original)

Foucault's work (1979) also maintains that there is importance in paying attention to the diverse ways that people understand the distribution of power and the multiple sites of resistance to domination. In keeping with the above definitions and ideas about political activity, one definition of political activity for our purposes is purposive action, which helps to create and define a self or group identity, which then allows for individuals and groups to redress perceived injustices and grievances. This definition helps to open up new spaces between the public and private realms, where many of the activities of the women fall. Thus, the definitions of community work that have been referred to in this section combine with the idea of informal politics. I strategically use the terms *activism, community work, politics,* and *political participation* throughout the book to denote the range of activities that fall within the informal political realm. In doing so, I am offering up a richer, theoretical space in order to explore the suggestive contour of women's involvement as political actors.

INTERSECTIONALITY

I argue that women prior to their HIV-status, occupied social locations that disadvantaged them and made them vulnerable to multiple stigmas. This situation created a qualitatively different set of experiences for the women, as compared with other people who contracted HIV/AIDS. The HIV/AIDS virus acted as catalyst, which made them recognize and act on other aspects of stigma in relation to their identity. The concept of intersectionality and stigma are tied together to form "intersectional stigma," the framework used in the analysis of women's participation. Intersectional stigma, it is argued, affects identity, resources, and participation.

Perhaps the biggest problem political scientists, and other social scientists encounter when trying to study politically active marginal women or women of color or both (and other types of women on the social periphery) is the difficulty in capturing the degree and role of intersectionality and intersectional experiences.

There are two strands of intersectionality, and the concept of the intersection of race, class, and gender as it has developed within various feminist theory literatures, which concern us here. The Intersectionality of experience in society, has been a driving theoretical focus, beginning specifically with women-of-color theorists trying to create relevant theory about the concept of multiple oppressions (see hooks 1981, 1984, 1989; Lorde 1984; Davis 1981, 1989; Dill 1979, 1983; Giddings 1984). Multiple oppressions, it is argued, can combine and create new and (often) unrecognized forms of discriminatory encounters in everyday life.[17] Moreover, intersectional experience suggests that one's social location is determined by the ways in which disparate oppressive conditions come together to foreground or highlight experience (Collins 1990; Hurtado 1989; King 1988; Smith 1987). Originally, many of these critiques were aimed at white feminists, who, it was argued, had obscured the experiences of women of color by positing gender as the *only* explaining locus of oppression or the most *consistent*, and *salient* one for all women. Similar critiques also arose from scholars engaged in separate areas of inquiry. These ideas mushroomed out across the academic arena due to their theoretical usefulness for exploring a nexus of questions about history, identity, and experience (see Andersen and Collins 1992, Haraway 1988; Harding 1986; Higginbotham 1992; for critical race theory and other jurisprudence see Crenshaw 1989; Williams 1991). These critiques reinvigorated feminist theory and captured the attention of theorists in many disciplines. Scholars reexamined central tenets in feminist theory through the prism of intersectionality, including experiences as diverse as labor, rape, sexual violence, and motherhood. Intersectionality has been sometimes called a metaphor, a methodology, a set of relationships, as a corrective to either/or thinking, and at other times as an analytical tool (see Andersen and Collins 1992; Brewer 1993; Chow, Wilkerson and Baca Zinn 1996; Zinn and Dill 1994; Collins 1995; Crenshaw 1997).

Concurrently, the second strand of intersectionality was discussed by Crenshaw (1989) in theorizing about black women's experiences within the law.[18] Within antidiscrimination law, she critiqued the legal system's ability to recognize discrimination of black women. She argues that compartmentalizing experience—either focusing on race or sex—diminishes the usefulness of the law and is a detriment to black women. She argued that this single axis type of argument is replicated in feminist theory and antiracist politics. Detractors and skeptics of intersectionality argue that the concept is difficult to model quantitatively, and it is theoretically not always feasible to explicate multiple sites of oppression (see Daly 1993).

Some critics see intersectionality as arguing for smaller and smaller subcategories or for nonsensical mathematical models (see West and Fenstermaker 1995a for critiques of models proposed by advocates of race, class, and gender analysis; for responses see Collins 1995; Maldonado 1995; Takagi 1995; Thorne 1995; Weber 1995; Winant 1995).

In response to these criticisms, Collins has argued that intersectionality is a willingness to see multiple sets of constraints and freedoms as an organizing frame for experience in U.S. society. Collins has labeled this idea as a "matrix of domination" (1990). This is a move toward understanding how *all* people are affected by this matrix and can occupy multiple and overlapping positions of oppression. Scholars have also stressed that intersectional factors and experiences are multiplicative, not simply additive (see Chow, Wilkerson, and Baca Zinn 1996; Anderson and Collins 1992; Collins 1990; Daly and Stephens 1994).

Collins (1995) responded to critiques of additive models of inequality that purport to represent the idea of intersectionality arguing that concepts of intersectionality emerged not just from academic inquiry, but also through the trajectory of contemporary social movements:

> These links between theory and politics meant that, despite their historical differences, all three areas shared certain fundamentals. Each aimed to explain the links between micro-level experiences structured along axes of race, class, and gender, with the larger, overarching macro systems. Each reasoned that, if individuals could link their own experiences with oppression on a micro level with the larger macro forces constructing their social position, they could address some of the major social problems of our day. (492)

Single- or privileged-systems thinking (e.g., class over race) left much of the larger picture of inequality obscured. Collins notes that intersectionality is

> a model describing the social structures that create social positions. Second, the notion of intersectionality describes micro-level processes—namely, how each individual and group occupies a social position within interlocking structures of oppression described by the metaphor of intersectionality. *Together* they shape oppression. (1995, 492; [emphasis added])

These positions are often in contrast with postmodern ideas where gender, race, and class concerns are sometimes recast as "performances," "interactions," "parodies," or as "simple subjectivities" (see Collins 1995; Thorne 1995).

In a recent work Crenshaw (1997) elaborated on the various ways intersectionality can be used to halt monocausal explanations:

> Intersectionality is a core concept both provisional and illustrative. . . . I hope to suggest a methodology that will ultimately disrupt the tendencies to see race and gender as exclusive or *separable* categories. . . . The basic function of intersectionality initially is to frame the following inquiry: How does the fact that

women of color are simultaneously situated within at least two groups that are subjected to broad societal subordination bear on problems traditionally viewed as monocausal—that is, gender discrimination or race discrimination? (552)

Crenshaw advances three different ways to understand and analyze intersectional experiences.[19] The first is structural intersectionality, or "the way in which women of color are situated within overlapping structures of subordination. Any particular disadvantage or disability is sometimes compounded by yet another disadvantage emanating from or reflecting the dynamics of a separate system of subordination"—or phrased another way, "the material hierarchies" are relevant in discussing inequality (1997, 552).[20]

The second understanding of intersectionality Crenshaw advances is "political intersectionality," which refers to the ways in which political and discursive practices relating to race and gender interrelate, often erasing women of color. This seems more analogous to her original use of intersectionality in the law. She suggests that either/or propositions stressing either race or gender within a given context are not useful. The last variant of intersectionality is "representation intersectionality," which suggests that popular culture produces images and representations that "converge to create unique and specific narratives deemed to be appropriate for women of color." She argues that "the clearest convergences are those involving sexuality, perhaps because it is through sexuality that images of minorities and women are most sharply focused" (Crenshaw 1997, 554). She maintains these types of images are harmful purveyors of justifications for continued discrimination, violence, and abuse toward women of color.

These are useful ways to begin to operationalize concepts like intersectionality. Until recently, little attention has been paid to the intersections of oppression that many U.S. women of color face; oppression and discrimination are often different from the experiences of white women, relational to other women of color, and complex in the intersection and creation of gender identity (Crenshaw 1989, 1997; hooks 1984; Hurtado 1989; Collins 1991; Chow, Wilkerson, and Zinn 1996). Because there exist so few studies that attempt to explain women of color's political experiences in the United States, there are even fewer that attempt intersectional analyses on any level.

Intersectionality is important to the integral argument about politics this book advances. Respondents are primarily women of color who are former lawbreakers. It makes theoretical sense to want to think through the ways in which their understanding of HIV and experiences of HIV and their later participation would have some relation to the intersection of gender, race, and class. Women in the sample cannot be referred to as "women" without a complex understanding of the ways in which their social location differs from that of other types of female political actors.

Second, it is argued that because of their social location they were *primed* to experience a devastating form of HIV-related stigma. When they became HIV-positive, all of the positions they occupied—drug user, sex worker, poor woman, were already concentrated, or saturated, with a set of representations and assumptions about those subject positions.

With this population and many others, applying concepts of intersectionality can help to crystalize and reinvigorate avenues of social science research. Understanding the complexity that results from the intersectional experience of HIV/AIDS provides an example of how further research can be carried out. I now turn to stigma, its importance to my theory building and its relationship to marginality.

STIGMA AND MARGINALITY

Stigma is a *specific* form of deviance (Goffman 1971). Deviance is a broadly conceived concept widely deployed in sociological literatures (see Pfhul and Henry 1993). Stigma and the stigmatizing process, because they involve relationships of power and interaction, are a very useful concept for understanding how they might interfere with aspects of political participation for an individual or group. Stigma has restricted people's political and social participation (see Plummer 1975; Schur 1983, 1980; Pfhul and Henry 1993). As Pfhul and Henry note, the "social limitations imposed on stigmatized people go beyond territorial protection and extend into almost every facet of everyday life" (1993, 177).

Studies of marginality and powerlessness revolve around how groups of people are effectively shut outside the political system, not necessarily by formal sanction or proscription, but by social sanction (see Cohen 1993 on African American mobilization on HIV/AIDS issues compared to gay men's mobilization; Gaventa 1980 on quiescence and hegemony; Lukes 1974 on power). The question that might arise during this discussion is, Why isn't these women's participation thought of as an outcome of marginality? It could be argued that because the women belong to social groups who have had specific, long-standing problems with access to resources and power, those conditions should be a starting point for explaining and understanding participation. This group's marginality is apparent. Why the focus on stigma and, later, on intersectional stigma?

Stigma and marginality are co-related factors in describing group experiences of "outsiderness." But stigma itself is a rich and previously ignored concept as it relates to questions of political participation, affecting resources, access, and outcomes. Stigma informs our understanding at the individual and group level about informal mechanisms of societal exclusion. The realm of stigma constitutes what has been called a "language of relationships" (Alonzo and Reynolds 1995, 304). It also can provide a map for how outsider groups might be able to overcome specific barriers to participation.

Stigma, in this instance, is one of the ways people who are marginalized experience themselves and describes barriers that interfere in their attempt to participate.

Stigma more effectively describes the societal reasons behind the overwhelming negative experiences respondents have faced in response to HIV/AIDS. Respondents' experiences with stigma are rooted in specific cultural histories and ideologies; they are time, place, and context bound. The types of challenges they have faced are not just about belonging to groups without political power, although the women belong to relatively marginal groups in society.

Also, stigma once acquired is difficult to reverse or challenge. It may have "a temporal dimension in that they [stigmas] are ineradicable and irreversible as the terms ex-mental patient or ex-convict imply. In fact, stigma may follow us through the life cycle" (Alonzo and Reynolds 1995, 304). Stigma encodes itself into a person's psyche with the resulting manifestations, including shame, self-hatred, internalization of broader group values, and repressed anger (Alonzo and Reynolds 1995). Schur argues that stigma and deviance involve far-reaching evidence of political norms. He posits "deviance [as] an inherent political issue." He explains,

> By definition, since they are modes of devaluing and discrediting, the designation of deviance and the deviantizing of individuals involved the exercise of power and affect the subsequent distribution of power. (1980, 25–26)

Other authors have also commented on the issue involved in stigma, which is power: "Power relationships are central to stigmatization. Stigmatization is an exercise of power over people and a manifestation of disrespect for them" (Gilmore and Sommerville 1994, 1342).

Stigma also has the potential to affect resources. The resources that concern this argument are time, money, and civic skills. People who are stigmatized often have some difficulty in securing steady employment; they also tend to have less money (Pfhul and Henry 1993). Stigma does not necessarily affect free time. The development of civic skills, like education, are usually deterred or interrupted in a stigmatized person's life. Because stigma has the potential to make one the target of violence and causes one to be avoided, these factors frequently mitigate against organizing (social or political) with other people (both stigmatized and nonstigmatized).

Marginality is related to concepts of disenfranchisement, but has often been conceived as more institutionally based, with a focus on material resources. Cohen, however, in discussing marginalization leaves an opening for the development of research on stigma as it relates to the area of marginality and political processes:

> The process of marginalization, through which groups come to be identified and exist outside the central institutions and systems of relating in society, can occur through the implementation of any number of strategies. Marginalization occurs and is reinforced when A, in some sustained manner, limits or excludes B from gaining access to, substantially participating in, or controlling those societal mechanisms—institutions, ideology, and social relationships—that determine the life chances of B. While the tactics of marginalization are various in nature, they generally take on three interrelated forms: ideological, institutional and social interactive. (1993, 40)

The ways in which marginality has been theoretically developed are not linked with interactional or other conceptions of stigma that inform Cohen's category of societal mechanisms of marginality. But if we are to understand Cohen's assertion that strategies of marginality are "multidimensional," then it behooves us to place studies of stigma alongside and as evidence of *marginality*. Cohen notes: "To understand the true impact of a marginalized status we must search out the subtle ways in which inequalities are defined, maintained, and heightened" (1993, 60). Therefore, concepts of stigma and intersectional stigma are constructs that help illustrate features of marginality.

INTERSECTIONAL STIGMA

For some people, stigma has the potential to confer social power and to inhibit or curtail social power for others. Now, when we interlink the concept of *intersectionality* with the concept of *stigma*, we can use it as a way to illustrate the various ways women are specifically disadvantaged in relation to all phases of the HIV/AIDS virus. Intersectional stigma points to an understanding that women are not only *marginalized*, and socially situated (shaped by race, class, and gender), but that the category of "HIV-positive person" is loaded (from a stigma standpoint) with effectively negative perceptions about groups of people with the virus (e.g., drug users, crack cocaine users, prostitutes, lower-income women). Additionally, these negative perceptions are overlaid within the axes of race, class, and gender. Their experience of this disease illustrates the points of contact within structural realities of race, class, and gender *and* indices of stigma. Together, they have created a context for women's experiences. HIV-stigma compounded each axis of inequality.

Other researchers have suggested the HIV/AIDS virus compounds and magnifies other types of stigma:

> Although the stigma associated with HIV/AIDS is overpowering, individuals with the illness do not necessarily experience the same degree of stigma. Differentials in stigma experience can be explained, to a large extent, by variation in individual social identities and attitudes confronted in one's social networks and reference groups. (Alonzo and Reynolds 1995, 305)

Land also discusses the devastating effects of HIV and stigma for women of color:

> Although minority women with HIV come from various cultural backgrounds, they share many common issues and concerns. In general, they are the most isolated and least supported group with HIV and often experience considerable *social stigma*. . . . These women present a shocking picture of what can happen to a people disempowered because of gender, race, ethnicity, and poverty. These women suffer the *stigma* of a disease associated with promiscuity, illicit drug use, and death. (Land 1994, 359–60 [emphasis added])

The effect of the HIV/AIDS virus shifted respondents from marginal positions into a highly specific discriminated-against collectivity. The concept of intersectional stigma provides purchase power in explaining qualitative differences in the experience of stigma and marginality.[21] Intersectional stigma also begins to unpack why the history and trajectory of their participation looks different when compared to other groups who organized around HIV/AIDS issues.

There are four specific categories of stigma that women experience through their (pre- and post-) struggles with HIV/AIDS. The categories of stigma are drug use, sex work, sexual trauma, and the HIV/AIDS virus.

1. *Drug Use.* Crack cocaine is an incredibly stigmatizing form of drug use (see Inciardi, Lockwood, and Potteigier 1993; Maher 1992; Maher and Curtis 1992; Ratner 1993). Historically, women were often drug users, but in relative numbers to men, they were almost inconsequential (Inciardi 1993). The rise of female rates of crack cocaine use increased during the late eighties through midnineties. Some research has suggested that there existed similar rates of crack cocaine use and even HIV infection between women from rural areas versus large cities (Forney, Inciardi, Lockwood 1992). Despite these findings, I would argue that crack cocaine is associated with inner-city use. This does not mean that other groups of women are not stigmatized, but they are not immediately associated with drug use and prostitution as many of the women in my sample have been. One of the best ways I have seen this theoretically accounted for is by Austin (1992a), who discusses how stigmatized black women, in particular, have

no convenient narrative to explain deviant behavior. For example, they cannot fit into the "bad male gangster" image because that is an exclusively gendered identity within black communities with a history and ideology to support that framework.

As Campbell notes, "women who use illicit drugs embody both individual deviance and social failure" (2000, 1). In that representations of female drug users conjure up abusive, out-of-control, unfeminine, and unmaternal women, they are viewed as society's "spectacular failures" (3).

2. *Sex Work*. Sex work is considered by many as a deviant activity, and is also criminalized in the United States (except in brothels in certain counties in Nevada). The majority of the women of the deep sample were street-level sex workers and were subject to stigma because of their actions. As they were also crack cocaine users, they faced compounded stigma in relation to their experiences of both street-level sex work and survival sex.

The phenomenon of sex-for-crack exchange[22] transformed street-level sex work. Urban prostitution had historically been a consistent feature in the majority of U.S. cities from the early-twentieth century on (Rosen 1982; Hobson 1990; Mumford 1997). By the mid-to-late eighties, women involved in street-level sex work and prostitution represented a wide social and economic spectrum; some women were functional drug users and prostituted to make additional money; others were primarily there to make money and were not drug addicted. Some women thought of themselves as involved in semiprofessional or professional activities (Jenness 1993). These women were often able to care for their children and lead a semifunctional if stigmatized life. Street-level sex work was usually organized through one or more pimps, a person (usually a man) who watched over the women, bailed them out of jail, and set up a place for them to live.[23] With the arrival and widespread use of crack cocaine, leading frequently to addiction, "survival sex," involving bartering for drugs, became an increasing norm (Inciardi 1993; Ratner 1993). Use and addiction to crack cocaine often devolved into a crude and unequal bartering system, driving down prices for sexual services considered degrading and unacceptable by most of the women (drug users and non-drug users) and often driving out professional prostitutes. Tension between women from different backgrounds and worldviews occupying the same territory was not unusual (Maher 1992; Inciardi 1993; Ratner 1993). In the new urban landscape (and the resulting vacancies in the sex trade made by the flight of non-drug-using prostitutes), there was a new stream of women who were heavily addicted and who would sometimes undercut established prices based on local norms. The organization of street-level sex work and drugs changed spatially. The nineties saw the development of various places, often referred to as crackhouses,[24] where men could have sexual access to the women who smoked crack. Some women were not able to negotiate for better prices, leaving them more vulnerable to ridicule, abuse, and violence (Miller 1993, 1995).

As another accompanying phenomenon, often during extreme pharmacological addiction women (and men) became bolder and more aggressive during the time they are pursuing heavy crack cocaine use. During the 1990s, the combined interplay of drug use and sexuality was particularly pernicious. Prostitution was a feature of many urban communities (and many downtown areas identified as "red light" districts). Crack use changed the terms of the often liberal agreement to "look the other way" by either residents or law enforcement or both. If standard and organized practices of prostitution maintained a level of privacy and secrecy, crack cocaine and sex-for-drug exchanges were publicly bolder. Traditional prostitution with its secretive and its spatially enforced separation from the "respectable community" was undermined in this new era by this more public display of criminal exchanges. Crack use was a public affair. It often transferred the boundaries of sexual activity and drugs to public space—parks, streets, abandoned lots and buildings—in ways that were often shocking to community residents and others (Maher 1992; Wallace 1992).

America's already conflicting codes and norms about drug use, prostitution, and accountability were strained even more by the eruption of crack cocaine throughout metropolitan areas. The political response to massive crack cocaine use (in particular female usage), with its resulting prostitution and challenges to public health was a punitive one.

3. *Sexual Trauma*. The category of sexual trauma refers to childhood sexual abuse and trauma experienced by over half of the respondents of the deep sample. Although sexual abuse in and of itself does not compose a deviant category, it is included here because women specifically felt stigmatized for being sexually assaulted. They also often experienced stigma *within* their families of origin if the abuse was confronted. It was a theme of central importance to respondents. This category involves feelings of shame and self-hatred and is overwhelmingly gendered.

4. *HIV/AIDS*. The focus on stigma is theoretically rich as it relates to the HIV/AIDS virus (and the position respondents found themselves in during and after diagnosis). HIV imparts a severely formative and traumatizing type of stigma.

The effects of the stigma of the HIV/AIDS virus have created and reinforced axes of inequality for women (Patton 1994; Stoller 1998). The response to the HIV/AIDS pandemic scapegoated several groups, and this scapegoating diverted public discourse into the direction of an "us versus them mentality" (see Alonzo and Reynolds 1995; Gilmore and Sommerville 1994; Patton 1994). There is a large literature that explores different facets of stigma that people with HIV/AIDS and their caregivers face (see Alonzo and Reynolds 1995; Bennett 1990; Gilmore and Sommerville 1994; Kelly et al. 1987; Lawless, Kippax, and Crawford 1996; Herek and Glunt 1988; Quam 1990; Weitz 1995).

It could be argued having the HIV/AIDS virus currently acts as a "master status," overwhelming and eclipsing other aspects of an individual's identity. Authors posit that "[t]oday, one of the most powerful and harmful stigmas is HIV-infection and AIDS (Gilmore and Sommerville 1994, 1341)." The scope of the virus and its impact is a crosscutting and unifying theme among researchers:

> HIV and AIDS are manifestations of an extraordinary illness in terms of its potential for multidimensional stigmatization. . . . [As compared to other illnesses] HIV infection and AIDS are rather universal in their preponderant negative evaluation. (Alonzo and Reynolds 1995, 305)[25]

Weitz argues that a "large part of having [the] HIV disease is the experience of stigma" (1995, 268), and that "[t]he threat of the HIV/AIDS virus is continuous throughout all phases—pre-diagnosis and post-diagnosis" (268). Weitz makes the argument that stigma related to HIV is a consistent feature of the illness:

> Stigma is a concern during all phases of the illness, from before the diagnosis, when individuals must evaluate the risk of discrimination if they get tested for HIV, to the time when death seems inevitable and they must cope with the possibility of discrimination by funeral directors. (Weitz 1995)

The ways in which people understand HIV/AIDS is indicative of the pervasiveness of its stigma. Gilmore and Sommerville (1995) locate seven metaphors for the disease as manifested in *language*. They discuss several powerful socially constructed metaphors: AIDS as death, AIDS as punishment, AIDS as crime, AIDS as war, AIDS as otherness, AIDS as horror, and AIDS as villain (1994, 1351). Each of these metaphors conveys disturbing affirmations of prevalent notions about difference, deviance, and stigma.

The acquisition of the HIV/AIDS virus is stigmatizing and, as some would argue, will continue to be stigmatized despite different populations becoming infected, because it is primarily contracted through bodily fluids imparted sexually.[26] Sexuality in and of itself is often a stigmatized activity (Brandt 1985). Stoller discusses HIV stigma and the way in which it reinforces other aspects of inequality:

> That stigma may have been attached to AIDS and HIV primarily because of the marginalized social status of the majority of people with the disease. But all who are infected are tainted by it; it plays a "master role"—a role that dominates one's perception of others. In the US, gender and race also function as master

roles, generating distinct behavioral responses in others, regardless of other roles that the individual inhabits, including occupational status. (1998, 136)[27]

Gilmore and Sommerville have a slightly different understanding of how the HIV/AIDS virus compares to other epidemics including STDs:

> Stigmatization related to AIDS differs in some respects from that related to other STDs. In the past, STD stigma often *caused* the persons to whom it was assigned to be seen as separate from society and its dominant communities, and as belonging to one or more separate stereotyped, minority communities. Members of these communities were seen to be "polluted," morally corrupt, dangerous, irresponsible, etc. In contrast, already stereotyped and stigmatized communities have been further stigmatized by AIDS. (Gilmore and Sommerville 1994, 1349 [emphasis in original])

When we identify how the HIV/AIDS virus affected women in the United States, we can note that women on the very bottom of the social ladder have absorbed the majority of the stigma in relation to the HIV/AIDS virus. The women becoming HIV-positive in the last two decades are often women already considered *deviant* in some way. Women of color, drug-using prostitutes, and urban residents continue to constitute groups of women with some of the highest risks of infection who occupy the edge of the social periphery. From this we can surmise that as they were impacted with the HIV/AIDS virus, respondents were already positioned within a set of structurally deleterious social discourses, which would shape and determine aspects of their experiences with the HIV/AIDS virus. This argument does not, however, suggest that their experiences were predetermined or inevitable.

Patton argues that in understanding how the HIV pandemic is gendered, it is not so much about the question of the early invisibility of women that has caused major problems.

> Particular and specific ways of carving up the category "woman" into a series of women-who-do-not-count-as-women was fundamental to the original paradigm through which researchers, policymakers, educators, and the media first understood the AIDS epidemic. (1994, 2)

She documents how these paradigms often were inflected with race and class bias. As Sacks notes, the way in which "AIDS discourses" have developed over the past two decades has helped to reproduce *perceived* differences between groups of women and not their commonalties:

> AIDS discourses on women are overwhelmingly about women whose behavior puts them on either extreme of female deviance. One end of the pole are the prostitute, representing the apparently indiscriminate woman, and the pregnant,

HIV-positive woman, representing the unfit mother; at the other end lies the "innocent" woman—she who became infected by her dentists, or by the sole unsafe activity of her life. (1996, 60)

Two scholars writing from an Australian context elaborate on this idea of the Western representation of HIV/AIDS:

[T]he HIV-positive body is more often than not assumed to be male. Nevertheless, in a way reminiscent of earlier discourses surrounding syphilis, women living with HIV have been positioned as a potential source of infection. This representation has contributed to the widespread discrimination, with women being positioned as "dirty, diseased and undeserving." (Lawless, Kippax, and Crawford 1996, 1371)

When we take these categories of stigma and combine them with the understanding of intersectionality (identified as the interlocking forms of oppression, which can be identified as separate, singular systems, but whose explanatory is greatly enhanced when they are seen as interactive and interdependent on each other), what we have then is not a methodology or just a theoretical example, but a narrative relationship between the interaction of these stigmas and social structure.[28] The "piling up" of stigmas does not result just in a negative effect; it changes and transmutes the relationship between other aspects of identity and HIV/AIDS.

Moreover, the concept of intersectional stigma helps to highlight the area of sexuality as a powerful route of stigmatization—because the majority of the women acquired the virus through a combination of drug use and prostitution. Given the often degraded status of crack-using prostitutes that this research and others have discussed (coupled with representations in popular culture and news media), this route of HIV/AIDS transmission carries with it onerous stigma (see Berger 1998; Fullilove, Lown, and Fullilove 1992; Boyd 1993; Inciardi 1993; Maher 1992; Maher and Curtis 1992). Because the context of the HIV/AIDS virus for respondents involved assumptions of drug use and prostitution, consequently they were not granted the protection of "innocent victimhood." Their experience of stigma that incorporates sexuality, race, class, and gender helps us to ascertain their unique responses to HIV and their struggles en route to political participation.

Intersectional stigma also illuminates the ways in which respondents are represented in discourses that speak to the interactive oppressive conditions that work to silence, thwart, hinder, and preclude participation in larger democratic forms of representation, debate, and process. They are composed of multiplicative influences that can singularly be identified as specific sites, but which collectively are not reducible to any of these sites—it is the totality that creates the specific form of intersectional stigma. The cumulative and qualitative effect of intersectional stigma differentiates them from many other social groups who have the HIV/AIDS virus, makes their process unique. Studying this group gives an aperture to understanding the narrative relationship between stigma and political participation.

Let us turn now to research that supports the argument that paying attention to social identity in relation to stigma and HIV/AIDS is important. Grove, Kelly, and Liu (1997) in their qualitative work with white, heterosexual, middle-class women and their experiences of the HIV/AIDS virus, point to the specific ways in which social identity/location can insulate people from stigma. Drawing on the work of Bourdieu, the authors discuss social identity as a way to understand social and cultural capital. Their study suggests that because the women they interviewed were not identified with any of the risk groups associated with the HIV/AIDS virus, their respondents were often invisible to doctors as people with HIV risk (e.g., doctors would ask them, "Why do you want an HIV test? You're not the type of person that gets that disease"). Moreover, the women did not experience *any* social exclusion or isolation and only very low levels of perceived stigma. The research finds that because of their powerful markers of social identity (in this case race, sexual orientation, and class) respondents could represent themselves as innocent victims, become "invisible deviants," and remain blameless. Furthermore, the authors note that respondents "can reveal their stigma, but in doing so, they are neither discredited nor morally contaminated" (Grove, Kelly, and Liu 1997, 335). These are very suggestive indicators of the ways in which social identity can insulate against stigma, and evidence of the ways in which social perceptions about risk and disease structure experience.

Intersectional stigma also suggests that respondents' multiple levels of stigma *precluded* their political affinity to other groups. Intersectional stigma differentiates them from other politically organized and agitating groups within the HIV/AIDS social movement—including sex workers and the queer community (lesbians, gay men, bisexuals, and the transgendered). It also explains not only their positionality, but also their experience of politicization in relation to HIV/AIDS.

To strengthen my argument, I turn to two groups of people who were also affected by the HIV/AIDS virus—gay men, particularly white gay men, and sex workers. By discussing these two groups, I argue that although these groups were relatively stigmatized in relation to dominant communities, they did not have the experience of intersectional stigma due to their connection with preexisting identities, and they were able to access organizational resources that helped them in responding to the HIV/AIDS virus.

Gay Male Mobilization

From the beginning of the HIV/AIDS epidemic it was characterized as a white gay male disease. Gay men, although marginalized within culture, simultaneously were situated to be able to respond to the crisis. They possessed significant cultural capital and symbolic capital and were able to cast themselves as if not experts, then at least as legitimate speakers within medical and social discourses (see Cohen 1993; Epstein 1991; Stoller 1998). Additionally, as Epstein notes, most affluent gay men in various cities had access to doctors and medical resources (1991).

Although, women, drug users, and others were present within early findings of people diagnosed with the HIV/AIDS virus, they had less cultural capital and were ignored (Epstein 1991; Schneider and Stoller 1995; Stoller 1998). The way HIV/AIDS (was and sometimes still is) imagined is through a white gay male lens (Stoller 1998).

Gay men are stigmatized within society. They have in the recent past and present been institutionalized because of sexual orientation, faced relentless discrimination overt and covert, and have been harassed, assaulted, and killed. However, they tend to command influence within the gay community as a whole, and also within their own social and economic networks. Despite their stigma, because they are male, gay men have had access to more resources compared to other stigmatized groups (even in the gay and lesbian, bisexual, and transgendered community); this phenomenon has been well documented (see Cohen 1993; Epstein 1991; Stoller 1998).[29]

Despite societal prejudice, as they acquired HIV they were in a much better position to mobilize themselves. One factor that contributed to this was their ability to utilize a primarily male medical establishment (as well as gay male doctors and health professionals) and their own resources, and the ability to mobilize people from the standpoint of a shared group identity (Cohen 1993; Stoller 1998).

The organizing went into challenging the medical expertise of the health and medical establishment, challenging homophobia, and changing popular understandings of HIV/AIDS as a gay disease—and therefore unworthy of attention. Through organizations like ACT-UP, San Francisco AIDS Foundation, and the Gay Men's Health Crisis,[30] gay men were able to plan, strategize, and respond to the HIV/AIDS crisis. They had peer groups, professionals within the community, and a wide resource base. Indeed, what distinguished them from other disadvantaged groups were their "economic access" and resources that helped build an "indigenous community" (Cohen 1993, 277). In the past ten years these groups have been more responsive to the diverse needs of the HIV/AIDS community. That effort has come through the hard and tireless work by other groups on the margin.

These initial events of the nonresponsiveness that some white gay men faced from health officials were some of the first times that they ever experienced stigma or discrimination:

> This experience would provide the first stage of politicization and consciousness-raising for many who, through either not openly identifying as gay or having the financial privilege to build a life (the areas where they live, the places where they work; the friends they have; and the establishments they frequent), they had been able to limit their encounters with a hostile, homophobic society. (Cohen 1993, 271)

The argument being made is not meant to minimize the intensity of the discrimination and stigma the white gay male community faced. Nor is it my intention to suggest a stagnant, homogeneous experience that all white gay men faced in confronting HIV/AIDS. It is, however, to suggest that because of their male identify, rarely did they suffer the burden of multiple stigmas. If any group was structurally in a "good" position to respond to HIV/AIDS, it was the white gay male community.

The other group we turn to look at through their experience of HIV/AIDS, stigma, and organizing are sex workers. Because of respondents' background, one might assume that they would be caught in the locus of activity that marked several sex-worker organizations and spawned new ones regarding HIV/AIDS. This was not the case. They are stigmatized even within the sex workers' movement because of drug use and their involvement primarily in a street-level sexwork.

Sex Work and Mobilization

The mobilization of sex workers around broad-based civil rights and human rights is not an entirely new phenomenon (Delacoste and Alexander 1987; Jenness 1993; Kempadoo and Doezema 1998; Pheterson 1996, 1989). In the 1970s in Europe, and then in the United States, sex workers collectively organized and engaged in social protest (Pheterson 1989; Jenness 1993). It was the first time that sex workers began to challenge dominant understandings of what the definition of prostitution was and assert the concept that sex workers had the right to organize on their own behalf. Prostitution itself was transformed into a new political subjectivity (S. Bell 1994).

Prostitute activists focused on the visibility of prostitution, the scapegoating of prostitutes as social pariahs, and the changing of laws that heavily favored men (Pheterson 1989). Other aspects of social protest often highlighted the brutality of the police, and struggled for a redefinition of prostitution (and other sexual services) as a type of work that should be governed under civil rather than criminal law (Pheterson 1989).

Shannon Bell describes the consequence of the various stages of prostitutes' rights articulation:

> These two historical processes, the first of which involves the extension of democratic equivalence to prostitute women, and the second of which arbitrarily refused women's right to work as prostitutes, mobilized prostitutes as political subjects. It is the contradiction between the extension of democratic equivalence and the state's campaign against prostitutes that produces the prostitute as a new political subject. (1994, 105)

For many women involved in these activities (particularly white women) of the seventies and eighties, prostitution was argued to be a part of one's identity. The construction of prostitution shifted from that of social stigma and victimhood to a site of multiple (and sometimes contradictory) meanings that included pleasure, work, violence, autonomy, and self-hatred (see generally S. Bell 1994; Chapkis 1997). Prostitution from the vantage point of an affirmative identity is not currently accessible for many women, both active and nonactive sex workers.

In many of the early organizations questions about race, and specifically about women of color, were included in the analysis of harmful effects of racist structures[31] in sex workers' lives (Delacoste and Alexander 1987).[32] The overall role(s) of women of color in prominent positions of the major organizations is somewhat unclear. In terms of leadership and central roles in these organizations, it would be fair to say that women of color, though involved, were not as visible as white women.[33] Generally, urban women of color sex workers were not centrally organized or targeted. Women of color (who in some estimates make up the majority of street-level sex workers) have never been a visible force in the leadership. Drug-using women also had been relatively excluded from earlier movement organizing, and continue to occupy the bottom rung of the social ladder among sex workers (see Delacoste and Alexander 1987).

Because of the effects of race and class in many women's lives (especially respondents) it is not possible or desirable for them to claim a space of subjective identity around prostitution or sex work or both. Very few women see themselves through the sole identity of prostitute. Some did have a sense of semiprofessional identity around sex work. However, the women could not easily incorporate the language of claiming one's identity around prostitution, and then HIV/AIDS activism. The structural and cultural mechanisms and influence for such a movement were not in place. Although sex work has multiple and fluid meanings among the women, at the time they acquired the virus, few had a meta identity of sex worker to fall back on. Overall, urban women of color did not (and do not) often identify with earlier concepts of prostitutes' rights. This does not mean that they do not understand or struggle with the concept of prostitution in their communities. Rather, it means that the discursive space is different (and continues to be different) for these women (and others) than for primarily white and European women in the seventies, and who currently claim(ed) prostitution as an identity.[34] Former women of color sex workers/lawbreakers are not in the same discursive category as are white women.

The terrain saw a discursive shift in prostitutes' rights as well as material changes (see S. Bell 1994). In the 1980s, with the advent of the HIV/AIDS virus, prostitutes began again to be scapegoated as the infectious carriers of disease (Jenness 1993; Schneider and Stoller 1995; Stoller 1998). This was reminiscent of several earlier periods in American history. When this shift occurred, other types of organizing around civil rights and the continued extension of the rights of prostitutes as citizens began to wane. Consequently, as Jenness documents, sex workers and prostitute organizations and collectives had to fight on several different fronts at once as HIV/AIDS educators (S. Bell 1994; Jenness 1993; Stoller 1998). They did this for both their communities as well as for the often, more hostile wider community outside of prostitution.

Nancy Stoller discusses the new identity that competed for meanings with others, which shaped the category "prostitute":

> In organizations like Cal-PEP and its parent organization COYOTE (Call Off Your Old Tired Ethics), which were formed to advocate for and provide services to prostitutes, a new and anomalous role has been established—the prostitute as outreach worker or reformed native. . . . The AIDS crisis, in particular, has given new life to the redemptive identity of "ex-prostitute." . . . In this context, sex workers may subversively accept the identity of disease carrier in order to secure funding, to force a place at the policy table, and to enhance recognition of their expertise in the public sexual realm. (1998, 84–85)

Women of my sample were not able to translate their knowledge into organizational resources solely as sex workers. Additionally, although there have been some halfhearted attempts to organize women on the street, there have been no truly successful efforts, and indeed Michigan is a state that has no active sex workers' rights organizations. Additionally, in Detroit, when the earliest women had been diagnosed there existed virtually no literature on women and AIDS or general HIV/AIDS organizations. By examining some of the experiences of other groups, we can surmise that although other groups faced stigma, the degree to which they were able to organize was predicated on already established or emerging identities and collective resources.

What does a focus on intersectional experience tell us about the potential for political participation? First, it suggests that intersectional stigma can affect social and political participation. Using the concept of intersectional stigma, we can theorize the ways it affected how they perceived themselves during their discovery of the HIV/AIDS virus, what resources they had available to them, their to routes to participation, and how they rerouted or diffused stigma. For people with intersectional experiences of stigma, participation requires an analysis of and redirection of stigma. All of these factors have been overlooked by traditional inquiries on participation. As noted previously, any of the stigmas discussed has the ability to overwhelm identity. Until stigma can be redirected, it will continue to affect the life chances and political opportunities people face.

COMING OUT OF THE SHADOWS: STIGMATIZED WOMEN AND POLITICS

This book offers a political analysis of the participation of a select group of stigmatized HIV-positive women with an interpretative framework of intersectional stigma at the core. By understanding how stigma plays a defining role in the process of political consciousness, it offers different answers about what forms their participation takes and what barriers they face in staying active. Chapter 2 introduces the deep sample of women in the form of narrative bio-sketches. It provides an overview of important events regarding their drug use, sex work, and criminal activities prior to their acquisition of HIV.

Chapter 3 discusses the qualitative methods used to collect the total sample of respondents and the style of analysis. The pathway to participation for women with HIV/AIDS, which begins with the social conditions of the acquisition of the virus, is the subject of chapter 4. The process of life reconstruction is the main focus of chapter 5. It delves into the mechanism of life reconstruction that begins with recovery. Chapter 6 investigates the respondents' struggles with facets of gender identity as an important component in their later political activity. It also discusses the tangible outcome of their sustained efforts—a persona, or public voice, and a defining role of what it means to be an HIV-positive woman. Chapter 7 illustrates the range of political activities in which the women are engaged, and how the concept of blended and overlapping roles is a useful heuristic tool to understand the meanings women give to the overlapping spheres of community, political, paid, and volunteer work. The last chapter, chapter 8, is the conclusion, advancing the claim that this work generates a new collective story of women who have become relevant social and political actors.

## CHAPTER TWO

Women's Narrative Bio-Sketches

THIS CHAPTER serves to introduce the reader to the sixteen women's lives whose political involvement and commitments constitute the core of the research, and provides a compressed narrative bio-sketch for each woman. The broad sociodemographic profile presented here portrays a group of women whose lives before they acquired the HIV virus were often complicated, for many, by drug use, sexual trauma, family abuse, poverty, and poor educational opportunities.

The bio-sketches give an aperture into the various types of disadvantages these women faced *before* their HIV-status, thus providing the foundation for their experiences of intersectional stigma *after* discovering they were HIV-positive. For each woman, information about her drug use, sex work activities, substance abuse treatment history, criminal activities, and other illicit activities is discussed. Additionally, an overview of family sexual violence, family abuse, or family substance abuse is provided.

Despite their earlier harsh life realities, the majority of women have been able to use the latest hurdle, their HIV-positive status, as a catalyst in developing skills and abilities not thought possible before the acquisition of the virus. The acquisition of the HIV/AIDS virus forced a reconsideration and appreciation of other aspects of their identity that had previously not been a central focus.

It would be impossible to present all the information that makes every woman unique. I do hope, however, to illustrate and allude to the general "worldview" of each woman, as characterized by her insights about particular events in her life. The reader will meet these women and their individual themes again throughout the unfolding of the book.

The focus in many of the bio-sketches is on defining and explicating negative and stigmatizing occurrences and activities. This rendering is unavoidable because it sets the foundation for understanding aspects of their transformation over time and illustrates the hurdles that they faced as political actors.

Table 1 provides a quick glance at important demographic characteristics of respondents that are discussed throughout the rest of the chapter and book.

The women are grouped together in the political roles that you will eventually meet them in chapter seven, either as activists, advocates or helpers. Each role constitutes a unique contribution to their communities.

TABLE 1.
Selected Demographic Characteristics and Life Experiences of Respondents by Race and Ethnicity

	African American	Puerto-Rican	European American	Other
Household				
# Poor/public assistance		1		
# Working poor	3			1
# Middle income	10		1	
Education				
# Less than H.S.	1	1		1
# H.S. graduate	2		1	
# GED	5			
# 1–4 years of college	4			
# of Respondents with Children	8			1
Experiences				
# Family Violence	4	1		1
# Sexual Trauma before age 18	6	1		1
# Battered after age 18	4	1		
# Family Substance Abuse	7	1	1	1
HIV Diagnosis				
# Prior to 1992	5			1
# After 1992	8	1	1	

Via the roles, each woman has found ways to enlarge and support her understanding of the HIV/AIDS community.

ADVOCATES

Charlene is a soft-spoken, forty-one-year-old African American woman. When I met Charlene it was on a troubling day—she was worrying about her low T-cell count,[1] and had just received a call from her doctor suggesting she try one of the new HIV/AIDS medications. Charlene was an adopted child and stated that her adopted status troubled her as a child. She was a member of a family with nine other siblings and could not remember many good memories from childhood. With an air of resignation she recalled the atmosphere of the house of her adopted parents:

CHARLENE: *I guess you would call it a warm house. I guess they did the best they could do. They was older people. OK. So, I guess you could call it a warm house. I got everything I wanted. I guess that was the happiest part, I got what I wanted.*

She did not feel close to either one of her adopted parents. She did not want to be an "adopted child":

> I wanted to be like other families. Have a real family. I didn't want no fake family, and that [her adopted family] was like a fake family to me.

She started drinking at the age of thirteen. Her education stopped at ninth grade. She described school as "boring." Charlene considered herself a tomboy throughout most of her childhood and adolescence, a role that did not fit with the family's image of appropriate behavior for a "young woman": "All they knew is go to church and go to school and wear them long dresses and patent leather shoes, and all that other stuff." The emphasis on ultrafemininity conflicted with Charlene's sense of herself.

Charlene used drugs recreationally in her early twenties, snorting heroin; then she moved to shooting heroin, which she enjoyed:

> And the first time I shot it [heroin] was like I was in heaven. I likes this. Then I just got to the point, I just started mixing the stuff. Just staying high all the time.

Charlene had little experience with street-level sex work. Because of her heroin use, she often took up company with men who were drug dealers. For income, she participated in stealing hustles, many of which she initiated. The father of her child and husband supplied her with alcohol and was a consistent batterer.

Cocaine was also a recreational drug, but when crack emerged on the scene she began to heavily use it, and to engage in street-level sex work. Charlene's comments about crack cocaine's effect in her life mirror those of many other respondents: "It took over my life. . . . Even heroin (which I dearly loved) became a second place drug for me."

She had a son in 1985 and tried recovery for alcohol in 1986.[2] She described mixed feelings about the treatment center and alluded to how some teachers in public school will pass students along without the student knowing the basics: "They just pass you on to get you out of the way." Despite this experience in treatment, she came into contact with counselors who helped her make lasting changes regarding her alcohol abuse.

Although she does not attribute her change in attitude about her husband's physically abusive nature due to her time in recovery, after she came out of treatment, Charlene said she was less willing to tolerate his violence toward her.

> I guess, the feelings I had after I came from recovery as opposed to then [before she went into treatment], it was like I was scared of him. But then after I got out of recovery after I had him [points over to her son], or a little before I had him, I told him [the husband], you know, "You put your hands on me now, I'll kill you."

A counselor from the program continued to form her main support system, and with her help, Charlene was able to achieve some stability and stopped smoking crack. She found out she was HIV-positive in 1986. She described how she handled it:

> *[I] cussed the nurses and doctors out, and left the hospital and never uttered a word about it for two years.*

Charlene, like most respondents, thought of the HIV/AIDS virus as a white gay male disease. She says when she told her treatment counselor and friends she lived with that she had been told she was HIV-positive, the counselor said: "'Don't believe them, you ain't got it.'" Shaking her head, Charlene said, "She was just as dumb as I was." She went on to comment that her friend's response was typical of many in the substance abuse treatment field at that time. There was not any medical or treatment follow-up for her.

In two years time, she began dealing with her HIV-positive status. She now works for an agency as a substance abuse counselor. In the late eighties she was a pioneer defining women's HIV/AIDS issues in Detroit. She counsels men and women for both substance abuse and HIV; she has also spearheaded community literacy campaigns.

Valerie is a thirty-five-year-old African American woman. She is dark skinned, sports elaboratedly braided hair, and often wears a complementary purple lipstick. Valerie comes from a large family of seven brothers and three sisters. Born in Mississippi, she was later raised in Detroit.

She was another respondent who had difficulty thinking of or conjuring up any defining good memories from childhood; she answered blandly about a few Christmases that were "okay." Asking her questions about her worst memories from childhood elicited the following:

> VALERIE: *Some bad things? Oh, Lord. Being sexually abused. And so that's why I care not to talk about my childhood, because whenever I'm trying to think of something good, that always creeps in. So, and even though I talked about it, it's still painful, so I choose not to really go into childhood things.*

She tried to tell her mother when she was fifteen about the incident with her father, and says her mother "chose not to believe me." As an adult, Valerie said she discussed this incident again with her mother and forgave her. Valerie credits the therapy that she undertook during substance abuse treatment that helped her bring up and deal with many disturbing issues related to the molestation. She said prior to that, "I didn't focus on it."

Valerie described herself as a "mouthy" little girl and young woman. She completed the eleventh grade and had a child at the age of eighteen.

She used marijuana with family members in her late teens, and became a "weed head." She also used crack cocaine with them:

> *I really hadn't heard a lot about it [crack], and I didn't know that my auntie and her significant other were using, and they were smoking. And we were at their house and I had my weed. And they were smoking. I'm just looking, and I hit it [took a puff of crack cocaine] and it didn't do anything for me, so I just didn't think about it any more. And, I didn't really get addicted to crack cocaine until I was like 26. Yeah, I'd say about 26.*

Valerie went on to obtain her General Education Diploma (GED) and also pursued an associate's degree in business. Her drug use escalated, though she cited no particular reason. She stopped for a few years, but when her second son was about two years old, she started again.

By the time her addiction got unmanageable, her family life also had deteriorated. Valerie was involved with a man her mother thought was not a good influence (because of his substance use) in her daughter's life. Through court order, her mother received temporary custody for Valerie's kids, and threatened Valerie that she would apply for permanent custody. At that point, Valerie decided to enter into a residential treatment program for her crack cocaine problem.

After leaving her first treatment program, Valerie was clean for about six months. She got involved with a married counselor (whom she met at the treatment center),[3] and because she was not able to have a satisfying relationship with him, she quit her program and started using crack cocaine with neighbors. She also began prostituting at this point in her addiction.

A stranger raped Valerie in her home, an event that triggered a bout of severe depression and heavier drug use. Valerie said she suspected that she was infected with the HIV/AIDS virus then, but was not sure. She tested positive in 1991 and received no counseling. About this experience she said:

> *I blocked out the HIV-positive. When I started back getting high, I think the HIV had nothing to do with it. I think, at first, it was just not being able to deal, and I was going to jail, and shit was falling apart, and feeling sorry for myself. It was more about the kids than I think it was the HIV.*

After many more attempts at recovery, she was admitted into a program specifically for women with HIV/AIDS who are substance users. She says the HIV/AIDS virus is one of her "biggest motivators" and after two years clean she decided she wanted to pursue working on HIV/AIDS issues and improving the quality of life for women and men with HIV/AIDS. She likes the challenges of working with the HIV-positive population:

> *I work with men and women. I don't have a preference, I'm so close to men, so it makes no difference about the male-female thing. I like working with people who are in recovery. HIV-positive addicts who are in recovery. That's who I like working with.*

Valerie has a paid position that helps men and women who are newly diagnosed with HIV/AIDS. She also works in prisons on HIV/AIDS prevention issues.

Nicole is a big woman with a clear cadence to her voice. She holds the listener's gaze and has a distinctive raised scar over her left hand. She is African American, and is forty two years old. She usually ends a conversation or an interview with "Have a blessed day."

Nicole has three brothers and an identical twin sister. She described her mother as a businesswoman, property owner, a strong presence in her life, and someone who was "doggone independent." Nicole said her mother was always encouraging her even when she made a mistake. A mistake, to her mother, was Nicole's pregnancy at the age of sixteen. Nicole decided to have her son.

In her late teens, the father of her child introduced Nicole to marijuana. Nicole said this introduction to drugs contributed to certain actions and behaviors:

> NICOLE: *And I think that's one of the reasons why I got in the predicament that I did as far as being pregnant. Because it seemed like once I started getting high and everything, it was like I had this overwhelming desire to have sex. I really can't explain the feelings but it seemed like sex was so much more exciting while I was high.*

She did not complete high school, and began working instead. During the seventies Nicole used various drugs socially, including opium, marijuana, mescaline, and various types of prescription drugs. She occasionally engaged in sex for money and worked in various jobs—as a cab driver, waitress, or factory worker. She explained her enjoyment of the lifestyle: "I think I just wanted to be hanging out."

Additionally, she sold drugs like marijuana and, later, crack cocaine. She was introduced to crack cocaine through a male friend. During several interviews, Nicole talked about crack being more exciting than other drugs. This pursuit of "excitement" had serious consequences later in Nicole's life:

> *During the time I was on the pills and smoking weed. . . . nobody could ever tell me I was an addict. Even though I wanted to be high every single day, I would have never thought I was an addict. When I started getting high off of crack and doing the things I did for crack, that's when I realized that something was wrong with me. I was like, "My God, that's a bad drug." Crack was the worst drug that ever came out.*

To encourage Nicole to break out of her social context of partying, drug use, and selling, her mother helped her secure a house in another neighborhood. She also facilitated entry into the nurse's aide and home health care professions. Nicole enjoyed this type of employment and is professionally trained as a nurse's aide. She takes pride in her ability as a caregiver. She told me she came from a "family of caregivers." She thinks her caregiving background contributes to her natural rapport with people and her ability to deal with being HIV in a positive way.

Her mother's dream, of Nicole finding stability quickly, however, started to deteriorate after a patient gave her money to buy drugs for him.

She was diagnosed with the HIV/AIDS virus in 1991. She continued to use crack cocaine until her mother died. On her deathbed her mother asked: "Nicole, would you please get yourself together? Get God in your life, and get yourself together." Because her mother always had a significant influence on her life, Nicole struggled to live up to her sworn oath to her mother that she would get off of drugs and get clean.

Nicole went into treatment right after her mother's death. She did not do crack after that period, but continued to abuse alcohol after she was released from the program. She realized she needed a well-developed inpatient treatment program, and got admitted to one where she resided for eighteen months. After this time, she began building her own strong networks with HIV-positive women; she slowly became a pioneer for women and HIV/AIDS issues. She now enjoys being an "insider" in the political arena.

Julianna possess a raspy Brenda Vaccaro type of voice and hearty laughter. She is a thirty-seven-year-old African American woman. Her hair is highlighted auburn and she wears large red glasses. She considers herself a "straight-shooter," and is very forthright. She was born and raised in Boston and came to Detroit as an adult. The first thing she tells me about her mother is:

JULIANNA: *She was a little activist in her own right. She worked until I was about maybe 10. Then she stopped working, she got real active in her little community stuff.*

Although she uses the word "little" in her narrative, there is nothing but respect for her mother's activities involving both the struggle for educational equality and civil rights issues. She has three brothers, a sister older than she is, and a younger sister. Alcoholism was a specter in her family because of her father, whom she described as a "happy drunk."

Julianna was a very good student, doing well both in high school and college, and said she did not give her parents much trouble growing up:

That's probably why I got started late. I did rebel, I just didn't do it when I was a teenager. I was just always, just on this path, and I knew what I wanted, and I knew what I wanted to do, so that's what I did. . . . I mean I never doubted that path.

Her path for a long time consisted of being a "good girl" and meeting everyone else's expectations. She still struggles with that today. During her junior year of college, her mother died, which triggered several depressive episodes and a search for intimacy from other people. She considers herself as someone who "deals" with things with grit and tenacity. About this difficult period she recounted: "So I made it through that semester, which was relatively easy because I had a lot of social commitments." She described herself as popular and outgoing. She contrasted this self-definition with the period of her life later on, when she used drugs and became socially isolated.

During this same time she got involved with a man. In the interview she went on to suggest that by being involved with this man, she was also caving into familial pressure about the type of life she should have. I asked if after her mother's death, she or any family members pursued therapy individually or as a group:

> No. And that didn't help either. Because as a family we all came together then, and then everyone basically went their separate ways. And it was hard, because I was still in school, and I was left there. But from talking to my sister, I don't think they did either. Everybody just kind of dealt with it in their own way. It was like everybody was concerned about Daddy and that was it. So nobody would allow ourselves to heal. So, I just went home after that summer after I graduated. I just couldn't wait to see this man, blah, blah. His family lived in Chicago. So when he graduated, I came with him [to Detroit]. So I came here. A year after that we got married [intensely mocking herself throughout her description].

Julianna said she felt unduly pressured by his parents to marry their son. This was also complicated by the fact that Julianna was already pregnant. In hindsight, she saw the whole affair as a mismatch.

She took a job in Detroit with a weight-management program. Her husband started using rock and powdered cocaine casually with friends, and began bringing it home. He asked her if she wanted to smoke, and she said she declined for about six to eight months. Prior to this, Julianna indicated, she drank alcohol and occasionally smoked marijuana.

She tried snorting cocaine, which was also popular among his friends. She did not like it because it kept her awake. She discussed how her husband went through many trial-and-error attempts before learning how to "fix" rock cocaine properly. After he learned how to make rock cocaine, he introduced her to the pipe, and she said without hesitation, "I loved it immediately." One of the reasons why she said she took to it was because of the fact she liked smoking, especially cigarettes:

> And I was like, oh shit, I knew that it was a mistake. Because it was just, I loved it. I loved it. Then we started doing it [smoking crack] together, and just [spending] outrageous amounts of money [emphatically].

For two years, they smoked crack almost every night. However, they were still able to maintain their lifestyle. He worked full-time in a well-paying manufacturing job, and Julianna continued to advance in her place of employment.

When it was clear crack cocaine use was affecting her husband's physical abilities, Julianna became vary scared about his addiction. Because she moved to Detroit for her husband, she had few social contacts of her own there and was without intimate friends. When asked if she or they did crack cocaine with friends later in their addiction, she replied:

> *I felt guilty and ashamed. I felt like, what if somebody found out and looked at me, and said, "She's on drugs." No, no, no, no. I would never have told them [friends]. Because I had an opinion about people who did drugs, so I figured they had the same opinion of me. It wasn't good. So, no, I never told anybody. But I began to cut back, because it was scary.*

Her husband continued to spend more money, became physically abusive, and endangered their child's life on several occasions. Julianna decided that even though her husband was lost, she could help their son and herself. She filed for divorce. After the divorce, Julianna moved around a lot, and after about a year was very lonely. She continued to use crack on and off. She described her rationalizations for drugs at the time:

> *I wasn't a druggie, I just got high. I wasn't one of "them." And so I started getting high by myself. Then I started doing it more and more and more. Every Friday on the way to pick Trevor from the baby-sitter I had to stop and get some. Then I'd have to sneak, because I didn't want my son, you know he was getting bigger by now, right? And I didn't want him to know where I was going. And then it got bad. And I started spending job money, spending rent money, spending money for things, getting behind on bills.*

Although the divorce helped Julianna in some ways, she was not able to stop herself from engaging in addictive behaviors. Julianna stressed she was desperate at this time in her life; she decided to make a major move: "In an effort to save myself, that's why I left and went back to Boston. I just sold my furniture, my bedroom set . . . everything."

In going to Boston, however, Julianna found little relief. She kept using crack cocaine. After she realized that she was still addicted to crack, and with her family becoming more suspicious, she decided to move back to Detroit and live with a man she had met earlier while using drugs. He did not use drugs, and even though he was a womanizer, she thought he might be a good influence for her (and her son's) financial stability. After she moved back, Julianna continued to use crack cocaine and started prostituting.

She admitted that she tried treatment more for her boyfriend than herself, and relapsed less than two weeks out of the program. She lost custody of her son to the state, which was a devastating blow to her. She temporarily stopped smoking crack of her own accord when she found out she was pregnant. Julianna felt strongly that she did not want this child. Julianna's life was at a crossroads when she decided to get an HIV/AIDS test; she decided to get a test because of her former lifestyle, and the results came back positive in 1990. She also now had a daughter. It took many years for her to stabilize. She is currently employed in a position where she helps HIV-positive women and also volunteers her time for a number of women and HIV/AIDS community projects.

Robin is an African American woman of blue-black complexion, thirty one years of age, with deep set eyes and a muscular build. She is part of a large family, four brothers and three sisters. She describes her childhood as normal: "a childhood like jumping rope and hopscotch and running after ice cream trucks, and things like that." When asked if any siblings have had problems with drug use she replies: "No, I'm the bad seed."

Being a dark-skinned African American woman with nontraditional features, or devalued physical features,[4] she said she fought a lot in school because kids called her names:[5]

> ROBIN: *I thought school was all right except for the part that I fought a lot. You know, because I always had short hair, and I'm dark, so I was always called names by boys: dark hair, midnight, ET, baldhead, blackie. I had most of my fights with boys. It wasn't so much with girls, it was with boys.*

Because of her fighting and other unpleasant experiences, Robin got expelled and transferred from one school to another. In junior high school she began to skip school. By the eleventh grade she had ceased attending school altogether. She described herself as "shy" and said she used alcohol to enable her to speak her mind and more easily socialize. The two conflicting sides that make up Robin are the shy side and the side who is adventurous and gregarious. Robin started using crack cocaine in her early twenties. Crack cocaine use was an extension of her experimentation with drugs and desire to become more outgoing:

> *It was always an experimental thing for me. There wasn't no tragedy or nothing like that made me go into it. It was an experimental thing. Then once I started experimenting, I kind of liked it.*
>
> *Well, to me it was still new. I didn't know what I was looking for. I didn't know what kind of high to look for, how this was going to make me feel. So about the fourth time, I guess it really hit me. I guess by then, I was hooked good. But the first couple of times, . . . it didn't bother me.*

For her, feeling out of control came "four or five years later." Robin worked various odd jobs as a waitress, a babysitter, and neighborhood tutor. Her behavior estranged her from her family. She primarily smoked crack cocaine with a close girlfriend. She described herself as "fast"[6] during her adolescence, and therefore able to attract men as "sugar daddies":

> *I was always . . . on the men. I was fast. I was the last one on my period [out of her sisters], but I was a little ahead of my time.*

The exchange of sexual services for money was a pretty early feature of her adolescence, and she expressed that this experience did not bother her. When she started heavily using drugs, prostitution was another avenue of income for Robin. She also began to sell marijuana and crack cocaine for several dealers. She stated that she was one of the few people who knew when to tell a dealer not to supply her with more drugs to sell because she was becoming too addicted. Twice she was arrested for carrying drug paraphernalia.

During the interview, Robin also expressed conflict caused between her role in the community and her drug-using and drug-selling activities. She often "looked out" for children in her neighborhood and was concerned with their general well-being. She said it was hard to reconcile being active in the affairs of the neighborhood and then being only three or four blocks away from her neighborhood, where she smoked crack cocaine. She also expressed a sensitivity for kids, because she is unable to have them:

> *It's a problem saying no to certain things. Just senior citizens and kids . . . because I cannot tell a child no. Because like in my addiction days, if a woman came [to her house where crack was sold] and you got a child, I really don't want your child to be in my house, but I would stop what I'm doing to let you go get high, and look after your kid. A lot of people found that out and they just took advantage of it.*

She was diagnosed with the HIV/AIDS virus in 1996. She immediately sought drug treatment for crack cocaine and began changing her lifestyle, embarking on the process of life reconstruction and empowering herself. She has had two major relapses, one of which is discussed in chapter 6. Since then she has become involved in volunteering with a program designed for HIV-positive families.

Constance is a smooth-skinned, honey-complexioned African American. Her voice is very soft yet direct. She wears red lipstick and has a regal presence. At forty-five years old, Constance is one of the oldest women in the total sample. Constance was born in Detroit to a family of five. She was the youngest. Her father was a factory worker and her mother was a housekeeper. There was no memory of drug use in the home.

She grew up in pleasant surroundings, and her family was "well off." She was one of the only black families living in the suburbs where her parents were able to move. She had this to say about her childhood:

> CONSTANCE: *I was from a good and loving family. They gave me everything. Sometimes though, I wanted more.*

She finished high school and went on to college to become a nurse, her childhood dream. The sudden death of her father struck an emotional and financial blow to the family. She and her siblings had to alter their plans and work in order to support their mother.

During the seventies, Constance used alcohol and marijuana recreationally. After moving in with her mother and coping with emotional and financial stresses, a friend told her how she could make some "quick money." Constance stressed in the interview how she was familiar with the "good life" and did not see why she had to give that up just because hard times were upon her:

> *So I tried what you call prostitution. I worked on the reference of a few other girls. Oh, it was such fast and easy money. I've bet you've heard that a thousand times* [laughter from respondent and interviewer], *but then eventually I settled into having a few clients regularly. Mostly white men, we traveled and I went all over the Caribbean and the United States.*

She liked being a self-described "call girl," allowing her family to think of her as a travel agent. Constance was displeased though when her sister found out:

> *My sister wasn't fooled for long. She knew and threatened to tell my mother. I had mixed feelings about what I did. Not bad, but I didn't want my family to know.*

After swearing her sister to secrecy, her activities continued for a few years. After another three years, she decided to get out of the business and she went back to school and finished her nursing degree.

Constance's introduction to crack cocaine was not until she was in her late thirties. She had used cocaine recreationally with her husband (whom she married when she was thirty one). They had sometimes smoked cocaine together. After the breakup of her marriage when she was thirty-six and due to her growing isolation, Constance turned more and more to heavy drug use as consolation. She said that the loneliness that filled her was hard to dispel. She quit her job: "You know I didn't have anyone to talk to really, the kids were teenagers and gone most of the time, so before long I was out there going to the places to buy crack."

After one attempt at recovery, she stayed clean for three years. She discovered she was HIV-positive in 1994. Constance has been disgusted with the way she and others have been treated by the medical establishment. She draws on her nursing and other professional experiences in advocating for women with HIV. Constance always sees herself as a professional woman, a former nurse and someone who takes great pride in her ability to challenge medical authorities.

Billy Jean is a thirty-one-year-old African American woman with doe brown eyes who grew up on the northwest side of Detroit. The death of her grandmother when Billy Jean was ten years old devastated her. She intimated that many "skeletons" came out of the closet after her grandmother's death that served to shake the family.[7] She has two sisters and one brother.

She felt an extraordinary amount of pressure to "lead by example," even though she was the youngest child. In the first interview we talked about the tension she felt due to her family's expectations and criticisms of her. Over the course of several interviews there were many times where Billy Jean told a disjointed narrative about her childhood years. The narrative moves between one about competition between the good sister (her eldest sister) and the bad sister (her) to one of her as a "failed child." The failed child narrative is encouraged by the fact that Billy Jean often feels she let her family down because of her history of drug use and prostitution, and her HIV/AIDS status.[8] Caught between these two narratives is her own insistence that she never received love as a child.

During a second interview, her experience of past sexual abuse came up in the context of her family life. She was eleven when her father molested her. She went to her mother, and her mother did nothing. He also was physically abusive to the family. The following is indicative of his severity:

> BILLY JEAN: *He whipped me with a water hose so bad, I couldn't sit down for a week. My whole back of my legs, matter of fact, I still got scars from the water hose. They're not scars that blend out [sic], but I couldn't wear shorts, short shorts, and stuff like that because I was conscious of the scars.*

When answering a question about why she left school early, Billy Jean stated her early sexual development as a reason:

> *But school was not a problem, but then when I got old enough to learn how to fuck, I stopped going to school. I found something else to do.*[9]

The idea of her worth as a sexual commodity is a consistent theme throughout much of Billy Jean's life. She described her young adulthood as populated by older men who raised her self-esteem, taught her things about life, and provided her with a basis for love which she felt was lacking at home. An early miscarriage made it seem as if she was not going to be able to have children, which greatly depressed Billy Jean. To the extent that Billy Jean has identified with traditional ideas about what it means to be a woman (e.g., having a child, being married to a man, being a conspicuous consumer, and owning a large house); these ideas dominate and permeate Billy Jean's struggles. She often feels compared to her eldest sister, who possesses all of the traditional things society (and Billy Jean's family) values.

At first, in her late teens, crack did not make a big impression with her. She said throughout the interviews, "I could put it down." Slowly, though, crack became more a part of her recreational and social life, and over time she "went looking for it": "At first I could stop on my own, but

I always used an excuse to go back, like depression, or a bad relationship, or peer pressure." She discussed moving from 151s[10] to the crack pipe:

> *I could put it down but I graduated to a stem [crack pipe] . . . it took you to a different high. See with the weed, it took you to a mellow high. With the stem it took you to an extensive high.*

She was homeless off and on for about two years when her addiction became more than she could control. Later she became involved with a man with whom she also had a child, and stayed with him a few years hoping to build a stable life. She soon discovered, however, that he was a womanizer or "whore." She said, "He wanted his cake and [to] eat it too."

Billy Jean tried inpatient treatment, but stayed only little more than a month. She found out she was HIV-positive in 1993 while she was pregnant with her son. Billy Jean's personal struggles continued through the next few years. Her reccurring problems with crack cocaine and inability to commit fully to what I have called "the life reconstruction process," which is integral to later political activity, has hampered her activities on behalf of herself and other women with HIV/AIDS. She has fluctuated between being a helper and an advocate.

Activists

Cherise is a thirty-two-year-old woman, with close-cropped brown hair and large dimples. She is African American. She presents a cool demeanor and does not get easily flustered.

She has one sister and one younger brother. Although close to her father, she described his drinking as "excessive." Her father constantly entertained both family and friends and also sold marijuana. She began drug use at the age of nine. Thus at an early age, it became easy for Cherise to obtain marijuana for herself and friends. Providing marijuana helped her gain access to an older group of social peers.

Her brother's birth marked a difficult time for Cherise. Before her brother came along, she had been a favored child, and after his birth she felt he received preferential treatment because he was a boy: "He came along, and just bumped me out of the way. I just believe that's probably my worst memory. I hated that." Later in the interview, she spoke, at length, about her feelings of replacement:

> CHERISE: *He got the attention. We all got [attention], there was nothing that I asked for that I couldn't have. So, it wasn't necessarily material things, but he got the attention and the love I didn't. That I think I yearned for. . . . I was supposed to be the boy they*

were looking for. But I wasn't, I was a girl. So they had to try again. And when they tried again, they finally got this boy that they wanted, and he was the youngest and the only boy. You know, and I felt like, they just like scrapped me to the side, and embraced this new person. And I felt left out.

She said that although her brother and she are close now, and though they even confronted their mother about the gender differences in her treatment of them, it was still a problem growing up.

She dropped out of school in tenth grade, even though she was a good student and had many favorite subjects. Her mother's strictness and discovery that Cherise was sexually interested in girls[11] eventually contributed additional conflicts to the household. After running away several times, she was sent to a program for troubled young girls.

After completing the program, she made good on her promises to stay in school, but soon she became part of a crowd of people selling and taking mescaline. She became estranged from her family after she began smoking crack cocaine in her late teens and early twenties. Her first crack experience was through a peer. In the passage below, she uses the word "dope" to connote strong drugs. Up until this point, Cherise had primarily used marijuana, mescaline, and occasionally alcohol. The drug her friend asks her to try is crack cocaine:

A friend of mine called and said, "Guess what I just had? It's so good." She said it was like freebasing only better. And I said, uh-huh. That's for—real dopers, you know. I was doing weed and taking a little mescaline, taking a drink, whatever. That ain't no dope. But you know, when you think about heroin and cocaine, to me that's dope. [Cherise says] Oh my God, girl that's dope. That's dope. So anyway, she called me up and told me, "I did this, and you just got to try it." And I'm like, shit, girl, that's some dope. I ain't going to try it. She said, "Just try it. Just smoke it one time. I just want you to know how it feels. And then you never, ever ever got to do it again if you don't like it." So I was like all right. So you know, actually I put it out of my mind, and then I was at a friend's house and I saw them smoking this, using this pipe thing. And I was like, damn, that's what Brenda was talking about. And so she offered me some and I was, like, OK. So I smoked some, and you know, I stood there like, you know, OK, what to do now? How long will it take? You know obviously I was supposed to be high then, but I didn't know what I was supposed to be feeling, so it was like it wasn't nothing. So I was like this isn't really nothing. So you know, every now and then I'd go over there, and every now and then they'd have some, and I'd smoke some, and it really wasn't about nothing.

Cherise's very circuitous route of drug use was mirrored by many respondents in the deep sample. Many respondents' early use of crack cocaine was casual, and it took a while for them to feel the more dramatic effects of the drug. Often they thought this drug was like other drugs—fun and controllable.[12]

She became romantically involved with a woman who was a heavy crack cocaine user, which contributed to Cherise's growing addiction to crack cocaine. This involvement also led to the beginning of Cherise's criminal activities. During this time she also began street-level sex work. She was arrested numerous times for soliciting and flagging charges.

Cherise discovered that she was HIV-positive in 1995. This fact depressed her and she continued using crack cocaine. Later in 1995 she sought treatment. Being pregnant and trying to find treatment was a difficult task.[13] She recounted a humiliating incident when she had to beg a treatment program director to admit her in; several other programs had already turned her away because of her pregnancy. She was incredulous at the level of hostility she received because she had no insurance. To the program director, Cherise said, "I can't believe that I'm here, poor, starving, no money and all you can think about is getting paid insurance."

A caseworker from social services came over to the program and asked Cherise to sign a form—Cherise contends, to this day, she did not know what type of form she signed. She was admitted to the program and able to stay in the program until after her child was born.

She has primarily been involved with outreach to HIV-positive lesbians, particularly those of African American descent. She is in the final stages of getting trained as an official HIV/AIDS counselor and also finishing a video on women with HIV/AIDS.

One of the first things that Shenna tells me during our interview is: "I'm probably not like the other women you've interviewed." What makes her unique is her style of activism.

Shenna is a twenty-five-year-old European American woman. She has dyed red hair, freckles on her face, light green eyes, and is slender. Shenna is an only child and grew up in a suburb outside Detroit. Her home life was "quiet." She said her parents were overprotective, and her father had a drinking problem. During the end of high school she met and dated a man two years older than herself. She says of him, "I got hooked up with a man who was all right." He often took her out to clubs in Detroit; she thought it was fun dating a "partyer." Shenna stated she noticed that he liked to drink, but it did not make a bad impression on her. She finished high school and had plans to go to college.

Shenna said she believed in the "happy ever after tale" about weddings and marriage she was told as a young girl. She married her now ex-husband when she was nineteen. She described their first couple of years of marriage as "okay." She delayed going to college. Because of his job they moved into a Detroit neighborhood, which Shenna did not like. His drinking increased. They often socialized with his friends in Detroit. The social circle they hung out with used powdered cocaine, and occasionally rock cocaine.

When asked about her first impressions of crack cocaine she said: "I didn't think anything of it when I first saw it. I was like 'is *this* what everyone on the news is talking about?'"

Shenna and her husband had talked about having kids. She became pregnant when she was twenty-two. Although she still had plans to go back to college, she was swayed by her mother and others' encouragement to have the child:

> SHENNA: *I talked about it with my mom, and because I didn't know what I wanted to major in, she stressed I have the baby first. I thought to myself, I'll just have this one, and then I can go do what I want to do* [emphatically].

She suffered an unexpected loss when she miscarried five months into the pregnancy. This event triggered a severe depression for Shenna. She indicated that during this time period her husband was not emotionally supportive of her:

> *He just pretended it didn't happen . . . like I was going to try for another one right away. His family acted that way as well. They didn't think about how hard all of this was on me.*

During this same period of time she noticed his drinking was becoming excessive. One night he brought home rock cocaine for both of them to use, and she liked it. After that episode, a year later, Shenna found herself calling up her husband's friends and trying to obtain crack for herself. She and her husband often used crack together. When they had to move from their apartment because of financial difficulties, she moved in with her parents. Shenna had many conflicts with them:

> *They knew something was wrong. I was hardly ever home, I borrowed their car to go into Detroit, which they despised. It was just a mess. I weighed so little during that time I got scared.*

She began prostituting in Detroit after she tried crack cocaine. She was diagnosed with the HIV/AIDS virus in fall 1995. She immediately sought inpatient treatment for six months. After this, she also spent some time with a close cousin in Minneapolis. She attributed this time away as very useful to her recovery and her ability to deal with the HIV/AIDS virus. She filed for divorce. This was a painful yet necessary process for Shenna:

> *He's still caught up in the drugs and drinking. I don't want to be stuck. I have enough challenges to face as is. I was really young and stupid when I got married. It wasn't the fairy tale everybody made it out to be.*

When she came back to Detroit she got involved with local women's HIV-positive support groups throughout the greater Detroit area. She proudly calls herself an activist and produces confrontational art.

KITT: *My [older] sister would call the school and say I had to come home. I'd come home and then I'd help her hit it [help her with setting up heroin works].*

Early in the interview, Kitt commented on the troubled nature of her childhood. "I was always near drugs and prostitution, that was always a part of my life . . . and my surroundings." Kitt is a dark-skinned, thirty-three-year-old African American woman with welcoming eyes and a soft voice; Kitt was born and raised in Detroit. Her father had an industrial job and her mother volunteered at different charities. Her mother drank often, and Kitt experimented at a young age with her mother's alcohol cabinet. She has eight siblings.

Kitt attributed much of early unhappiness to her older brother sexually molesting her. He was twenty-seven years old, and she was around ten or eleven when the molestation first began. After she told her parents, who did not believe her, her brother started physically abusing her. She believed her parents protected her brother because of his long-standing involvement with the neighborhood church. She said she could not take his rage and abuse, and left the house for good when she was eighteen. Kitt explained that there was a lot of drug use and chaos in her house. Most of the siblings used some type of drug. From an early age, she was involved in helping older siblings with their drugs (heroin), either helping them to obtain it or helping them to use it. The majority of her siblings abused heroin, and her parents "allowed it to happen."

She declared she went to "the street of Woodward. Woodward Avenue and became a prostitute at the age of thirteen." Kitt was an outcast and "never felt loved." Although she went back to her family's house a few times, she could not endure the family's rejection of her.

Kitt expressed that due to the traumatizing nature of her early experiences on the street, she routinely self-medicated with alcohol and marijuana. Kitt said she "often did things I didn't want to do just to have a place to stay." As she grew up on the street, when she could she worked out of bars and restaurants. She soon met a man who was a traditional pimp. He took her under his care and introduced her to another woman whom he also took care of in a traditional pimp/prostitute relationship. The three of them periodically traveled to different states, and he arranged paid sexual encounters for them. This experience defined Kitt's early teen years.

The two of them introduced her to snorting cocaine. She used many different types of drugs in her teens: heroin, powdered cocaine, mescaline, marijuana, and opium. Kitt's usage of crack cocaine came later, during her twenties. A sister introduced Kitt to crack cocaine on one of Kitt's occasional visits to her family. She used off and on, and then was able to stop, and even stayed a year clean without treatment. Her mother died during this period, and she said she felt "guilty" for never being around. Kitt would occasionally visit her family and spend money on some of them, still trying to gain acceptance.

Kitt complained that often women who smoked crack cocaine were belittled and treated poorly; their sexual services were driven down in price. She has observed what other researchers have documented (Maher 1997). She felt women were more vulnerable on the street. Seeking to avoid being in a vulnerable position, Kitt tried to generate income in other ways. Kitt came into contact with the criminal justice system many times, being picked up for stealing, forgery, and counterfeiting money.

Crack cocaine took a large toll on Kitt because as she explained, "This was the first drug which I *had* to do everyday." After three years of smoking, Kitt tried to commit suicide because she thought she "couldn't stop"; after the failed suicide attempt she then sought substance abuse treatment.

During the time she was clean she obtained her GED and also began training as a medical technician. While doing outpatient therapy in 1995, a psychiatrist (after finding out about her sexual and drug history) asked for her to be tested for the HIV/AIDS virus. She was tested, and when the results came back positive, Kitt said she was given a pamphlet and unhelpful comments by a doctor. She could not pay for insurance or available treatment. Kitt went back out to what she knew—to the streets. This incident, as it did for many other respondents, contributed to heavy substance use. She said it took her another few months before she was able to accept it.

The brother who molested her was a heroin addict and died of an overdose. When asked how she felt about that event, she said, "I didn't have no feelings." At her brother's funeral, she went up to the casket and said: "You're finally gone. I'm happy." She said that it has been a struggle for her to learn to love herself and work through childhood pain and trauma. Throughout her time in dealing with HIV/AIDS, she has concentrated on core issues stemming from her childhood.

Kitt has worked with agencies (and independently) to provide street outreach to homeless women and has conducted what she calls "rough house" HIV/AIDS prevention and education. She talks to young women on the street, giving them information, about both anti- and proprostitution organizations, if they want to stay "in the life." She feels strongly that if women want to be "professional prostitutes," they need to have several types of services available to them. Overall, however, Kitt encourages women to leave the "life." Kitt is also determined to have a nursing degree.

Daria is a thirty-seven-year-old African American woman. She has a rich and heavy voice, and almond shaped eyes. She grew up primarily in Detroit. Her maternal grandmother raised her. She has three sisters and one brother. Daria has happy memories of her father driving in a cab with her and also of being taken to his barbershop. Despite these pleasant memories, Daria noted that her father was an alcoholic and she described most of the men in her family as "drunks." She began drinking at around the age of seven.

Her uncle molested Daria from age four to about fourteen. She said she did not tell anyone because she thought that it was "normal," and that is what "uncles" did. He gave her candy and money and took her out before and after the sexual encounters. Although her mother told her to stay away from him, Daria says her mother never openly brought the incidents up. They also moved around the time of her late teen years. She suspects her mother was molested by someone in the family as well, possibly her uncle.

Daria described herself as a rebellious kid. She felt her mother could not keep her "safe," and she said, "to hell with everything." Daria dropped out of school in the ninth grade. A girlfriend introduced her to a wide variety of drugs. She said although she did not like any of them, she kept using all of them steadily. When asked why, at first she shrugged her shoulders, and then said, "I needed something at that time in my life." She said during this time she "went straight to the streets. . . . I became a hooker."

She originally thought of being on the streets as obtaining "fast money, easy money, and money to support myself." She traveled across the Midwest and to New York. She said that during that time she encountered pimps in the traditional sense, but thought it was repugnant to give her money over to a man. She alternated between thinking of prostitution as a professional career and as an activity she did not want to do. Like some other women in the study, she had sex work experiences beside the street level kind. While she lived in California she gained experience working in a massage parlor and escort service for several years. She had this to say about working in a massage parlor:

DARIA: *That was cool! Free drugs, the money was much better, it was safe. . . . You didn't take no chances, you didn't have to deal with perverts . . . Only perverts in another sense.*

Daria worked in California for five years. She met other women like her who were "in the life" as sex workers and recreational drug users. She suggested her drug use at this time was moderate and mostly recreational. She actually started using crack cocaine in California. She stayed there until about 1987. When she came back to Detroit, her drug use temporarily slowed down. She began using crack cocaine again after the birth of her first son. Crack changed how she thought of prostitution. She had previously used it as a way to support herself—not a way to solely support her drug usage. She used crack heavily. By her second pregnancy, she was very unhappy with her life:

I was depressed. I didn't want to have another a baby and my whole life was shit. I was hooked on something I didn't know how to get off of. . . . I didn't know why I kept running back.

Daria checked into an inpatient residential substance abuse treatment program for sixty days, and stayed clean a year. Soon after she began dating a man. She told a long story of being convinced to marry this man with whom she had been occasionally romantically linked. He did the "convincing." When I asked her why she used the word "convincing" she said:

> *I didn't want him to marry me. . . . Convince me—because it was more like security. It's not what I wanted because I wasn't happy with him.*

He also convinced her that she was "cured," and did not need any more treatment programs. He suggested she "just drop treatment" and settle into the role of wife. They got married. Within a few months she relapsed after three solid years of a combination of inpatient and outpatient programs. She said everything in her life grew worse.

She tried to commit suicide, and went into another treatment program after that episode. After two months, she relapsed quickly and also found out she was HIV-positive while in prison in 1991. During this period, she went without treatment for another year, and after being released she did more drugs and says she "really got high." She gave over custody of her kids to the state. Daria was finally admitted into a rare and special program for women with HIV who are in various stages of recovery.

During the first several sets of interviews I conducted with her, she was worried about the reactions of peers to the news that she was HIV-positive. "You get rejected a lot," she said often. She described one family incident in detail:

> *My sister was downstairs and I went and opened the refrigerator to get some juice. And she came running upstairs, and gave me a plastic cup. And then later I used one of her cups and she said I could take it with me.*

Since telling her family of her status, Daria said of her family members, "there are no more hugs and kisses now." Daria said the best thing about being HIV-positive is that it has "kept me away from drugs." She discussed how coming to terms with having HIV allowed her to find out different things about herself, including the strength to deal with her early childhood molestation. She said that previously she really disliked men. "I think about men . . . I tried to use them before they use me."

In repeated interviews, Daria stressed she wanted to be a productive citizen. On the urging of another woman in early 1997, Daria began her own support group for women with HIV who have been molested. She said of this experience: "At first I was depressed talking with other women. But we have so much to learn from each other."

Recently Daria finished her GED and has had difficulty in making a transition from a lifestyle of "easy" money to more stablility. She would like to go back to school to become a social worker. Her main focus is helping women (both HIV-positive and non-HIV-positive) to get in touch with their sexual traumas, including incest, rape, and torture. She is an emerging activist around sexual survivor issues.

Helpers

Cynthia is a tall, stocky, dark-skinned woman with pearly white teeth. She identifies herself as "other" because she is Jamaican, Indian, and black. She is forty years old and came to the United States as a child. Her mom came to the United States to work as a domestic and later as a nurse. A foster grandmother, her mother's first employer upon coming to the United States, primarily raised Cynthia. Cynthia has two siblings, a sister and a brother.

Cynthia has a twin sister with whom she was very close during childhood. When her mother remarried, there was family trouble and turmoil. Her sister was taken away and sent to live with another family member; her brother and Cynthia stayed with her mother and stepfather. Cynthia said this event shook her very foundation, and she alluded to the dramatic portrayal of the separation of two sisters in the movie *The Color Purple*:

> CYNTHIA: *I was devastated. We were like; have you ever seen The Color Purple? We were like that. I mean, that whole thing, crying, everything, the whole scene* [emphatically].

They are not close now.

Her stepfather raped her when she was eleven. When Cynthia told her mother her stepfather had attacked her, her mother did not believe her. Furthermore, her mother did not take her to a hospital after the incident. Cynthia said her mother just

> *cleaned me up in the tub and whipped [me] all while she was cleaning up. And my whole uterus to this day is still messed up because of that [the rape which she was not treated for].*

Her stepfather also physically abused her mother, and her mother would drink heavily after they fought. The rape, the continued sexual molestation, and the impact of her mother's abuse triggered Cynthia's exploration of drinking and taking pills (primarily over the counter) at an early age:

> *And it was like, my mother, every time my mother would leave or go to work, he would come chasing me around, and scare me, beat me down and tell me, "If you tell, I'm going to kill you, I'm going to kill your mama, and I'm going to kill your brother." And I just was scared to tell. Then that's when I started taking a whole bunch of pills. I found out that my mother had liquor hidden somewhere in her room, because they slept in separate rooms. And I used to go in her room and drink the liquor, and take pills and stuff, and just fall out and go to sleep. By the time my mom come home, then, she didn't do nothing, didn't say nothing.*

Cynthia describes her home life during this period as "stressful" and suggested it affected her schoolwork and ability to achieve her educational goals. Her mother told her to "just close your door," and directed Cynthia to put clothing trunks against the door to deter her stepfather. Cynthia spoke at length about how unsafe she felt in her own home. During this same time, Cynthia befriended a family in the neighborhood; the mother helped Cynthia relocate to the south for a brief time. Cynthia described this as a brief but happy period in her late adolescence. Unfortunately, this peace was short-lived. Several white men raped Cynthia and her girl-friends. The rape left Cynthia pregnant. One of her close friends never recovered from a coma she suffered from after the attack.

Cynthia had mixed feelings about having the child produced under such terrible circumstances, but had been "drilled" early on by family members that abortion was a sin. She decided to have the child and returned home to New York. She describes her pregnancy as sparking the closest bonding time between her and her mother that Cynthia had ever experienced.[14] Other family members raised her son. She never maintained a rapport with him, and he died while in college.

Cynthia's substance use quickly progressed from alcohol to heroin. She dropped out of school. She alternately divided her time between prostituting and working as a secretary. She expressed difficulty in dealing with men in romantic situations because of her many unresolved feelings about her stepfather. She described her early notions of prostitution as "revenge" on men, in that they would pay to be comforted by her, but she had no feelings for them. For about two years, she traveled with the money she made as a self-described "call girl." About these experiences she stated:

> It was a job. It wasn't to me it wasn't just prostitution because I wasn't walking the streets. I had people that hooked me up, and I had it in my little phone book of how much money this person would give me, and that's it. And I had my money limit. I didn't want nothing under a hundred dollars. He wasn't going to get the whole works for less than hundred dollars. Back at that time, for me, I was a high-class call girl . . . Black, but I wasn't walking no street. When I got to the drugs, really, really to the heroin, and then the coke and crack, I started mixing them together, then I started getting a little tacky. I started mixing with drug dealers.

After drifting through jobs and occasional heroin use for a number of years, she got involved in a supportive church community on the East Coast which helped her get back on her feet. Cynthia has always felt a strong connection to church and religious service, and possesses much religious or spiritual fervor. As will be explored later, this religious/spiritual faith is a resource Cynthia frequently draws upon to help other people. Her sense of a religious connection allows her to construct her expertise to "speak" truth to people—the truth of divine insight.

She continued to have serious bouts with heroin and drug use, and began smoking crack in the late eighties. By this time she had moved to Detroit. She got very sick while working as a nurse's aide and got tested for HIV in 1990. She tried outpatient recovery several times. Throughout her narrative on the road to recovery she speaks about the influence of spirituality in her life. This is mirrored in her approaches with people with HIV. Her participation has included spearheading HIV/AIDS projects within churches. She works with young people, and is also a spiritual adviser.

Shelly is a petite, mahogany-brown woman with curly hair usually styled in a bob. She talks very quickly and has several nervous tics, including repeatedly touching her hair and face. She is a thirty-seven-year-old African American.

She was born in Detroit and grew up on the east side. Shelly's family consists of three sisters and a brother who was deceased by the time of the interview. She identified some of the best times during her childhood as the times when she and her siblings traveled with her father. Memories of her mother are much more disturbing to Shelly. Her mother was an alcoholic. She often left the house after a period of drinking, which would cause arguments with her father. Her mother routinely left the children alone, drank excessively, and sometimes began relationships with other men.

She described her childhood as a series of negative and frustrating attempts to get her mother's attention. Shelly often stayed outside looking for her mother and getting into trouble, figuring if she was bad, maybe her behavior would prompt her mother to come back home. This strategy brought many experiences to Shelly, but did not prompt a significant change in her mother's alcoholism.

"Fast" is a word Shelly used repeatedly through the entire interview to describe her early sexual experiences. Shelly recounts a long history of family sexual abuse throughout her narrative. She attributed her sense of sexual knowledge to the fact she had so many sexual encounters, consensual and nonconsensual.

After she had a child at fourteen, her mother got her life together, stopped using drugs, and became a minister. Her son was born blind and with other mental and physical disabilities. Because of Shelly and her boyfriend's ages, the child's father's family claimed the child and raised it. Shelly was stripped of parenting privileges. This was very upsetting to her. Shelly indicated that while growing up, people often thought of her as "slow," but she reassured me that she is a capable, functioning adult. Regarding her son, she said both families "treated me like I was his sister."

Often Shelly talks about herself in terms of a good girl/bad girl dichotomy and suggested her upbringing was sheltered in some ways. This theme will reemerge later in chapter 6 during her narrative on her life reconstruction. Shelly graduated with a high school diploma and moved in with an older man; she knew this man off and on during her young adulthood. She stayed with him until she was eighteen and then got a job. Her use of drugs began as a recreational activity, and then moved into dependence, primarily due to her involvement with her older lover:

SHELLY: *I started drinking beer and liquor with young girls [who were] about fifteen, I was twelve. And then they introduced me to him, and I started smoking weed with him.*

At the same time she became an "acid head." About her relationship with the older man she stated: "He controlled my life, and I didn't know that, until I got thirty years old." She suggested he controlled her life by telling her what to do and when to do it. He monitored her recreational drug use:

But then he started telling me he didn't want me to do it [drugs] without him. And then, he made me do it every now and then with him.

She describes his kind of abuse as also having an emotional dimension: "A little before we broke up, he told my mother that he would make sure nobody else ever had me." Shelly's experimentation with many different drugs, including crack cocaine, progressed. After a disastrous period of crack cocaine use she entered a residential treatment program. It did little for her addiction.

Boredom was a big factor in her ability to stay clean. She said she could not afford to get "bored" once she had been on drugs. Since she was considered a "good girl" by some growing up, there were a lot of men in her community who wanted to become intimate with her when she decided to become a prostitute. She described a humiliating process:

That's all the guys wanted to do, they just wanted the opportunity that they've been trying to get since they've been kids . . . because Shelly didn't mess with nobody. I was a good girl, until I got twenty eight, twenty nine years old. You know and that was their first opportunity. "Shelly's getting high . . . we got it going on. She's giving [it] up almost free" [delivered angrily].

When asked what contributed her wanting to leave the lifestyle, she recounted how she was raped and stabbed by a male client[15] with a screwdriver twenty-seven times. During the interviews she showed me the wounds.

She discovered she was HIV-positive in 1994. She volunteers her services at Participation and Partnership for Health.[16] She spoke at length about the time it was taking her to recover and heal from almost twenty years of destructive relationships and drug abuse. She works on community HIV/AIDS prevention issues geared toward young people.

ANNA: *I've been an alcoholic, I've been a crack head, I've been a prostitute, you name it. I've been a fighter. I've been to jail. I've had a pretty rough life.*

Anna possesses a smoker's raspy voice. She is a forty-one-year old Puerto Rican American with long, dark hair who also describes herself as "Hispanic." There is a large scar over her eye from a previous fight with a current partner. Her troubled childhood was marked by death and sexual violence: "I was only five years old when my mom committed suicide. And she left five of us. I got two more sisters and two brothers, and we've been separated."

Her dad and other male relatives abused her beginning at the age of seven; her father was also an alcoholic. After being passed among relatives in Puerto Rico she became sexually active and was sent to the United States. She described herself during the period she lived with her aunt as a "slave"; she treated Anna as a live-in maid. During her time in the United States she went from using alcohol to speed (methamphetimene), powdered cocaine, and then rock cocaine. She usually used drugs with male partners. She said this of crack:

Once you get on crack, it's really hard. I do not wish on nobody to get hooked on crack because you will do anything. You will rob, you will kill. When you need a hit, you can smoke, you can smoke one time, you can smoke a rock. Then you turn around, all you want is more and more and more. There's no stopping it.

Anna got pregnant at fourteen and also had developed an addiction to alcohol. She tried recovery twice, both times for alcohol. It was difficult for her to remain sober:

I don't know. It's probably the people, you know, coming back to the same neighborhood, you know. Not really having a place to live, because I didn't. But I didn't tell them that, or else they wouldn't have let me go. You're supposed to, you know, when you go into treatment or something, they should make sure that people know . . . make sure where they're going to stay after they get out of treatment because if they're going to be running around up and down, they're not going nowhere.

She found out she was HIV-positive in 1995, and has since been active in HIV prevention; she organizes meetings and outreach programs for the Latino community in Detroit. She still, like Billy Jean (though for different reasons), struggles with the alcohol and drug dependency that has interfered with her ability to stay active consistently.

Simone has large eyes, high cheekbones, and a broad smile. She is African American, forty-one years old, and was born in South Carolina. She left South Carolina and came to live with her aunt in Detroit around the age of fifteen because her mother was fatally shot by a family member. She never knew her father. She has two brothers and two sisters. Simone described her childhood in South Carolina, "as good and with a lot of love."

Simone's troubles began when she lived with an aunt in Detroit whom she described as "color struck." She went on to say her aunt preferred light-skinned blacks. She was treated differently from her other cousins. Recounting her relationship with her aunt elicited a lot of emotion from Simone during our first interview. Simone believed she was not shown love by her extended family because she was considered dark-skinned.

The urban environment was a new one to her; Simone said she missed the outdoor activities that she used to do in South Carolina and felt limited in her new urban landscape. Although she liked school, she said she enjoyed it primarily because it kept her away from home. She dropped out of school when she was in the tenth grade.

She began hanging out with some girls who lived in the neighborhood. They introduced her into "the life." This was primarily defined as drinking, smoking marijuana, and hanging out at bars. She was introduced to older guys and began to experiment with heroin. Her aunt asked her to leave her house when Simone was seventeen. She said she moved in with a man and in a year or so they both had developed small "habits" of heroin use. She says of her involvement with this man, soon "all hell broke loose." He introduced her to the streets and when money was slow, he asked her to prostitute. Simone did not like working the streets, although she had engaged in casual paid sex before with a neighbor.

As her habit progressed, she wanted less and less to share money or drugs with her boyfriend. She went out on her own and says she became more "gritty and selfish" about her drug use. She worked out of bars, hotels, and restaurants during the seventies and eighties. In Simone's late thirties, a girlfriend introduced her to crack cocaine, and she immediately liked it. She described her crack addiction as ravenous, changing her character while she used it: "There was no limit to what, or who, I would do to get that drug."

After being destitute and going into a treatment for both heroin and crack cocaine, she was asked if she wanted an HIV/AIDS test back in 1990. She consented and found out she was HIV-positive. For another two years she went back to using drugs intensely and then found out about Nicole's group in Detroit.

After two years had passed, Simone was leading an HIV-positive women's support group that she structured and designed. She is also involved with helping high-risk pregnant teens who use crack cocaine and getting them prenatal and other types of care.

Georgia is a loquacious, funny, and warm woman with a heart-shaped face. She talks nonstop and occasionally snaps her fingers. She is one of the older respondents in the total sample, and the oldest of the deep sample. Georgia is fifty years old and identifies as African American. She comes from a large family of nine brothers and she is the only daughter. She grew up in Minnesota and came to Detroit as an adult. She could not tell me what her happiest memory was as a child because:

> GEORGIA: *I was always an adult and never a child, because you know, at ten years old, I took care of babies, fixed breakfast, you know. Got kids off [to school].*[17]

Her family was very financially secure, owning a rooming house and a small grocery store as well as having a father who worked in the steel mills. She talked about the combination of having to be an adult, coping with her father's rigidity, and being overprotected (by her father and brothers) as a window into why things "went wrong" for her. Additionally, being almost raped by a man at a young age and not having anyone understand or believe her experience traumatized her.

Georgia conveyed that she always, but especially early on, had an ambitious drive. "I wanted to be one of the first black women engineers or business administration or marketing people. I'm excellent with math." She returned to this description of herself as good with numbers and business, which she attributed to her "success" with criminal activities.

Her ambition was squelched when her father tried to restrict her in high school and told her she could not attend her high school graduation or participate in graduation ceremonies.[18] While discussing how upset she was about her father's behavior and his strictness, she simultaneously discussed how she perceived how women were treated in her community:

> *I seen how men treat women, and I didn't want to be a part of that kind of life. I wanted to be independent. I always wanted to be independent.*[19]

Although Georgia, did not come out and say specifically in the interview that her dissatisfaction was because of unequal gender arrangements, it can be inferred from her narrative that she was concerned as a young woman with how to get power for herself. Her reasons for starting to get into a lifestyle that would help her economically was also a rebellious attempt to get her father's acknowledgment that she could survive without him:

> *I started because of the things I wanted to make my father see that I could do it, too. If you won't help me, I'll do it on my* own [emphasis hers].

She continually talked about her attempts to attend college, "to go to school," and how farther and farther away she got from that elusive goal. Her late twenties were marked with a marriage to a man who would later become her criminal partner. Her husband was abusive throughout much of their time together. Georgia sold hard drugs throughout most of her adult life.

She discovered she was HIV-positive in 1995 when she was in prison. She considers herself a poet and a "real life educator." She has advocated on behalf of women with HIV, but also uses the arts and entertainment as a way of getting people to explore the issues of HIV. Georgia conveys tensions within her own life in her work in HIV prevention with high-risk kids. She has also periodically used her organizing skills in support of the other HIV-positive women's projects.

Life Lessons

This descriptive chapter has laid the groundwork for understanding the context of women's lives prior to the acquisition of the HIV/AIDS virus, also providing a brief summary description about the types of participation that the women became involved with after becoming HIV-positive. We have a beginning and hints at an ending; thus subsequent chapters will fill in the very important middle of the story. Before moving on to those dramatic moments, it is critical to highlight the degree of similarity across respondents' experiences and what it might suggest to us regarding wider patterns for stigmatized women with HIV/AIDS.

Most of the women suffered familial abuse and over half of the respondents also suffered sexual abuse as children. Other respondents were exposed to sexual trauma and violence outside of their family of origin. There is research suggesting a connection between sexual violence and later exposure to HIV/AIDS (see O'Leary and Martins 2000). Cuccinelli and De Groot also argue that sexual violence determines HIV risk exposure for women and girls:

> Sexual violence puts women directly at risk for HIV infection, and the emotional and behavioral sequela of sexual violence may indirectly escalate their risk of HIV infection. Women who are survivors of childhood sexual abuse are vulnerable to HIV infection because they may become involved in abusive relationships or may exchange sex for love, drugs or money. . . . Women who have a history of childhood sexual abuse are also . . . more vulnerable to HIV infection because they are more likely to prepare themselves for sexual intimacy by drinking or drugging. (1997, 225)

Often the trauma women experienced was not believed or validated. Respondents carried that stigma and psychological discomfort for many years. During life reconstruction, respondents are able to get direct help with the emotional experience of trauma.

Most women had trouble concentrating in school or left school early or both. Thus, respondents were without the structural and material benefits that educational achievement provides. They may have been labeled as troubled, unruly, and uninterested children, which also might have predisposed them to be ignored by instructors. Some respondents, then, had neither a stable home nor the "disciplining" effects of an educational institution. Thus after leaving school their choices as workers were severely limited. Some were condemned to participate in low-wage economies. Moreover, due to the lack of educational attainment, respondents were often left without other ways to participate in informal drug economies except through sex work and survival sex. Additionally, the vulnerability that women face in the crack cocaine economy has been extensively documented (Inciardi 1993; Maher 1997). Charlene, Robin, and Georgia are exceptions in that they worked closely with men and participated in other illicit income-generating activities outside of sex work.

Respondents' associations with men very often determined the emotional and financial structure of their lives. Their descriptions of men/relationships/marriages mark time and measure the women's own lives for them. Also, often a woman's drug use is connected to her romantic/emotional life. Women are frequently introduced to drugs through male peers. In my group, however, female peers and family were also just as likely to introduce a young woman to drug use.

Crack cocaine is not usually the first substance used or abused—but usually follows alcohol, marijuana and other drugs. This supports other findings of women's patterns for substance use (Maher 1997).

Cherise, Georgia, and Charlene expressed dissatisfaction with the range of gendered expectations they experienced in their families. Their response to these expectations and constraints was unique but provides an important aperture into the gendered patterns of many women's lives.

There is a cycle of drug use, recovery, relapse, and drug use that some of the respondents become trapped in. Many respondents were caught in a loop that included trying to remain clean, dealing with primary childcare responsibilities, recovery, and substance abuse. They also received gendered language about their roles and expectations of them as mothers that also contributed to feelings of shame. During this time the public discourse around accountability, motherhood, and drugs reached a crescendo, often polarizing women in the middle (Campbell 2000). Respondents often did not have the structural or emotional support (especially if they were mothers) that enabled them to stay drug free.

Finally, the context of the HIV diagnosis provided an interruption to this destructive cycle, adding a dramatic catalyst to their lives. This cycle of drug use, occasional sex work, and later HIV infection should suggest to us that there are not just individual choices at work in the lives of many women who find themselves less than satisfying options.

When looking at their lives collectively, one could also argue that society failed some of the respondents' early on with the lack of safety, comfort, and material advantage that ostensibly could have been theirs if they had been born into another social class or for some another skin color.

The other ways that society continued to do a disservice to many respondents was to make it more difficult to obtain substance abuse treatment and adequate care, especially for those who had children.

Furthermore, I suggest that in contrast to white and/or middle class women (who use illicit drugs or engage in illicit activities), usually poor and stigmatized women of color who use illicit drugs are more likely to be targeted and subjected to punitive bureaucratic state-sanctioned penalties (loss of child custody, discrimination from the medical establishment, criminalization and imprisonment, loss of social service benefits) (see also Campbell 2000; Maher 1997; Roberts 1991; Silliman, Bhattachrajee, and Davis 2002; Zerai and Banks 2002).

My hope in the presentation and analyses of these bio-sketches is to offer a continuum of respondents' experiences and familiarity with "the life." Moreover, in this discussion, I am reminded of the sage insights that Campbell (2000) makes when examining other feminist drug ethnographies or qualitative research on similar topics: "Explanations that rely on individual deviance marginalize the systematic and everyday aspects of drug use and addiction" (202). She argues that ethnographic insight on stigmatized female drug users frequently operates within a form of realism and that "they effectively reinforce existing power relations, social antagonisms, and divisions." (204). Respondents offered up a diversity of opinions about drug use and the role it played in their lives. Some respondents embraced a more "pharmacological" rationale about their crack addiction (e.g., "I couldn't control myself because of this drug"). Recall, however, that several of the women did not know what high "to look for" during first uses of crack cocaine, suggesting that drug use is also about cultural expectations in addition to the "real" effects of any particular substance. And despite popularized notions about the "addictiveness" of crack (the one "hit" makes you an addict notion), many women were not immediately addicted to crack cocaine.

Although the ravages of poverty, homelessness, violence, and sexual trauma have complicated their lives, we would be remiss if we did not remember the complexity that women bring to their own understandings of agency, pleasure, victimhood, and victimizing. I have highlighted by necessity some of the more difficult and somewhat depressing points of their narrative. But, there were many times in their narratives that "the life," HIV/AIDS, or drugs did not dominate the interview. While often feeling discouraged about particular life events, respondents also displayed creative responses and strategies of resistance to the circumstances that they found themselves in. Ultimately, if we focus only on the "deviant" aspects of their lives or note only the lack of strong social control of institutions and families, we miss how women build, as Pettigrew (1997) suggests, "self-defined lives" that go beyond traditional investigations.

## CHAPTER THREE

Capturing the Research Journey/
Listening to Women's Lives

IN THIS CHAPTER I review the methodology that informed my approach to the writing of this book. I characterize throughout that the process of the women's participation as a journey; so too was the research for me. I was involved as a witness, seeker, recorder, researcher, and narrator of their conditions. The outcome of this journey for me is a sustained commitment to help explicate the insights stigmatized women bring to their understanding of politics. I used multiple methods (a combination of life history and oral history approaches, ethnographic fieldwork, and observation) to obtain the oral narratives on which to base my analysis. Each method helped clarify and bring into focus aspects of the women's lives. Section One discusses the multiple steps I took to gain access to the women, and section Two discusses the process of analysis.

This is a comprehensive accounting of the key components of methods including the process of fieldwork, the interviewing of respondents, coding, and analysis. The first section concerns itself with recounting how the actual gathering of data about female lawbreakers evolved into questions about stigmatized HIV-positive women's political activities in Detroit, which is the central focus of the book. The second section explores the range of interpretative issues in researching stigmatized women.

Researchers have tried to find appropriate metaphors for the process and verisimilitudes of qualitative research, in particular, the ethnographic experience (see such diverse accounts as Geertz 1973, 1983; Abu-Lughod 1988; Anderson 1990; Behar 1993; Maher 1997). The ability to illuminate such a distinctive process often requires an appeal to the senses and to metaphorical language. Researchers struggle to convey not merely the mechanics of these experiences, but to capture how they arrived at knowledge about their respondents (Hammersley and Atkinson 1983).

SECTION ONE: FINDING THE WOMEN

Constructing the Study Sample

In the course of my research, I officially interviewed sixty women and informally observed the lives of a dozen more. Sixteen of the sixty women are HIV-positive and constitute the *deep sample*, and the focus of the book.

These sixteen women were the only ones, I believe, in the overall sample who were HIV-positive during the time of my research.

The *entire* population who participated in this research shared two similarities: they all had a self-defined problem with crack cocaine and had some experience with sex work. This net was initially cast wide in order to fulfill three basic goals: understand the meanings women attach to crack cocaine use, explore women of color's participation in street-level sex work, and investigate male violence toward female drug users. As I discuss in detail later, my research interests grew to incorporate an analytical snapshot of HIV-positive women crack cocaine users through active use, recovery, and empowerment that include a wide range of activism. Among my specific techniques for identifying respondents were self-identification, snowballing, chains of referral, and theoretical sampling.

Gaining Access and Defining the Field

When I first entered the field in Detroit I was filled with loathing, fear, and dread. Some of these feelings were characteristic of someone just beginning fieldwork—as evidence of an uncomfortable process where nothing is familiar and the researcher is introduced to new norms and behaviors. In the qualitative literature this process is typically referred to as "gaining access" and "getting into the field" (Goffman 1989; Hammersley and Atkinson 1983; Feldman, Bell, and Berger 2003). At the onset of fieldwork the researcher must recalibrate herself or himself into a new "sense" instrument—you learn in context about your new environment, absorbing new smells, sounds, body language, speech, and codes of behaviors (see Hammersley and Atkinson 1983; Burgess 1982). Contributing to my sense of discomfort was my feeling of being "sentenced" to what I considered the worst city in the United States. I had been to Detroit several times, and had formed negative opinions about it.

Detroit has been described as a metropolis that is not a city or, rather, as a "post-industrial city."[1] As Herron argues in *AfterCulture*, Detroit occupies a special place in the American imagination as a "city [that] embodies everything the rest of the country wants to forget" (1995, 9). He frames Detroit as quintessentially postmodern because of its modernist tale of success, enfranchisement, and the promise of the American dream that marked it during the powerful rise and development of the automotive industry. The subsequent decades of decline and its magnitude has raised the question, What went wrong in Detroit?[2] Through a cultural theory and poststructuralist reading, Herron suggests that Detroit can no longer stand as a symbol; it has been drained of its history. Like many other American cities, it functions as a physical space "where everything can be seen, but where little remains real," because it can no longer provide for its citizens (Herron 1995, 81).

In 1994, however, I was beginning research in a Detroit that had some hope generated by a new African American mayor whose political platform was designed to woo business back and ease racial and labor frictions. In addition, earlier in the year, several of Detroit's neighborhoods were designated as part of President Clinton's Empowerment Zones, which promised help with economic infrastructure. Governor John Engler had espoused renewed political commitment for various revitalizing projects throughout the city.

Locating Active Female Lawbreakers

During the summer of 1994, I went about trying to learn how to situate myself within the Detroit scene. I had very few practical ideas about working with stigmatized populations, specifically women who smoked crack cocaine and participated in street-level sex work, I was versed in the theory, but not in the nuts and bolts.[3] Initially, I used three strategies to meet women and become familiar with Detroit: one was volunteering at a woman's organization; the second was maintaining a field presence; and the third was talking with women at the Thirty-sixth District Courthouse.

I set out to establish myself as a credible person on the street, particularly in the Cass Corridor, an impoverished neighborhood in Detroit. This is an area with high incidences of drug use and street-level sex work, and high rates of poverty and homelessness. I volunteered with Females in Trouble,[4] a nonprofit organization sponsoring many programs geared toward community development and the self-empowerment of girls and women of the greater Detroit Area. Their services include a teenage homeless shelter, a mentoring program, and a Street Outreach Program.

To volunteer in their Street Outreach Program that serves many areas, including the Cass Corridor, I went through an extensive training program that was driven by the philosophy of Females in Trouble (FIT), which is supportive of women on the streets. They do not espouse an anti-prostitution agenda.[5] No overtures are made to reform or redirect them, but information is provided about leaving "the life." Help is offered in the form of many other types of services that women need, including obtaining important documents (e.g., birth certificate, social security card), drug treatment referrals, and domestic violence counseling.

The Street Outreach Program consisted of a van staffed with volunteers who rode around various neighborhoods in Detroit four to five times a week. They distributed condoms, bleach kits, hygiene kits, food, clothing, and blankets to homeless women, female drug users, and sex workers.

My shifts were usually three hours long. I familiarized myself with several areas of Detroit in this way, though I did not ask anyone for an interview while I was on my shift, nor did I knowingly interview any active FIT clients.[6] By learning about community services within the Detroit metropolitan area in this way, I was on a steep learning curve. My reputation on the street slowly developed because many women had seen and met me through my work on the van.[7]

Observation on the Street

During the summer of 1994, I maintained an active field presence in Cass Corridor, and also on Fort Street (a primarily Mexican and Mexican American area). To solicit women, I left discreet fliers at local bars, motels and hotels, particularly in Cass Corridor.

At first I allowed myself to be an observer, not asking women for interviews; instead I watched them as they obtained drugs and engaged in picking up men for "dates." The fieldwork shifts on several days ranged from ten at night to seven in the morning. Other shifts ranged from about eight at night until two in the morning.

I made contacts with people who vouched for my safety in the field, which allowed for free and undisturbed movement in the area. After my initial reactions to strong language and uncommon topics, I settled in to try to understand the context of women's everyday reality within the local street-level drug economy and milieu.

Court

After two months of intensive work in the field and through my volunteer activities at FIT, I met Carol Jacobsen. She is an award-winning cinematographer who made *Street Sex*, a video about women involved in sex work and drug use in Detroit; for the video she had solicited and interviewed her subjects outside the Thirty-sixth District Courthouse. This is the primary location where individuals of both sexes within the Woodward area are arrested, taken to court, and prosecuted for a variety of offenses, including soliciting, flagging, illicit drug use, carrying drug paraphernalia, and the like. After my meeting with Jacobsen, she suggested that I position myself around the courthouse, where I could meet women after they had been released. I decided this was useful advice, and began going to the Thirty-sixth District Courthouse.

After observing trial proceedings for many days, I was fortunate when a guard mentioned the daily HIV/AIDS Awareness workshop: when individuals are arrested for soliciting, flagging, or carrying drug paraphernalia, they had to attend an HIV/AIDS workshop as part of their bond and release. This workshop was held every afternoon at the courthouse.

The workshop had a guest facilitator from one of several agencies throughout the city, including Partnership and Participation in Health Organization, Hispanic Community Support,[8] and the Herman Kiefer

Detroit Department of Health. Counselors discussed safe sex and HIV prevention strategies and answered other questions about sexually transmitted diseases (STDs) for an hour. I introduced myself and described the nature of my work to the facilitators, and asked if at the end of the workshop I could say a few words to the participants.

During the period that I observed different people's response to the HIV/AIDS workshop, I noticed people were often bored, tired, or hungry; as the years passed the workshops became shorter and shorter. When I began my research they lasted for an hour. By the end of 1997 they were reduced to twenty-minute segments. Many of the women had heard the "spiel" about HIV before because they had been brought in many times on other charges. The men (not including transgendered male to female [MTF] people), who had been picked up because they solicited a sex worker, were distracted, sometimes overtly hostile, and often inattentive. They sat grumpily with hands folded squarely across themselves, sometimes with toothpicks edged in the corners of their mouths. Through their body language, they announced how inappropriate they thought it was requiring their presence at the workshop. Occasionally, someone would ask a sincere question, but typically male participants asked lewd questions, made sharp comments, or interrupted as if to hurry the speaker along.

Toward the end of the workshop, I would announce my work and take names and phone numbers from interested women.[9] I would always carefully explain to them that I was looking for women who were using or had used crack cocaine and had engaged in sex work.[10] Those were the two consistent and salient characteristics of all the women interviewed. Some of my first interviews came through the women I met at the HIV/AIDS Awareness workshop.

Throughout my entire research period I continued to return to the Thirty-sixth District Courthouse periodically because it was a rich source for contacting potential respondents and of indirect sources. My learning at the Thirty-sixth District Courthouse was heightened by the conversations I had with women's children, judges, bailiffs, treatment counselors, HIV/AIDS prevention people, and numerous ordinary folks. They all provided important contextual information about Detroit. After sitting for so long through the processing of various cases, invariably a lawyer, judge, counselor, bailiff, arrestee, or staff person would approach me, and ask me what my business was in the courtroom. I learned quickly that *everyone* had an opinion of the women they defended, worked with, arrested, counseled, and sentenced. Everyone had an opinion of how the situation with women and drugs had changed over the course of the past few years. Generally, bailiffs and other staff people were invaluable in helping me gain access to rooms in the courthouse, when I needed to conduct an on-the-spot interview and provided me with other types of privileges within the courthouse.

Creating the Deep Sample: Recovery, HIV/AIDS and Political Participation

> It didn't register to me until later that Penny is probably back on the streets. [Penny is a woman I interviewed in 1995 when I first began work with women in recovery. She didn't relapse until almost two years after I interviewed her.] I really liked her. I liked her energy, and her boldness. Not only when you find out people relapse your heart breaks, but intellectually you feel duped, cheated, used, a con, faked out, stupid, and betrayed. You want to really root for people, and you're never sure who's going to make it. So in this context, how do I go and re-examine my findings? Her narrative? Will I see her as "failed," a failure, the other, the unworthy? Will I carry my hostility and suspicion into the analytical context? Will I castigate her, or rub her out [of my memory]? Will I say this is the "one that got away"? Or failed? It's not personal—it's her life, her resources, her stuff, not mine.
>
> Now that is at least what I tell myself when I write my notes up. But it still is disheartening, even after all these years of working with women on the street. It's hard to set boundaries. (Fieldnote, April 1997)

RECOVERY

There is a common misperception in the imagination of the American public about drug use and recovery. It follows something like this: A person messes up and gets addicted to drugs. This individual goes to a drug treatment center, gets clean, and then returns to being a normal citizen. Right? The above entry from my fieldnotes, I think is illustrative of the chimerical nature of recovery in the lives of the women whom I studied.

Not only is the above hypothesis a naive assumption, it has little factual basis in the lives of the women under study or in other populations of recovering addicts. Recovery is a messy, ongoing, and tentative process. As some of the women I had interviewed during the study period decided to try to "get clean," it seemed natural for me to follow them through their experiences in treatment programs. Interviewing them in recovery was not always a conscious effort on my part. Sometimes, I would not see a woman on the street for a long time, and then months later I would run into her, and she would tell me she had tried some form of substance abuse treatment. I would often ask to interview her about her experiences in a treatment facility. Did she have support from her family? If she had children, where were they? Because of the multiple challenges women faced in staying drug free, treatment and recovery issues emerged as a compelling interest.

Although I take issue with the naive approach to understanding recovery, I admit that I, *too*, was startled to discover that, on average, recovery is not a one-time encounter for the respondents. The average woman in my group has gone to recovery at least *four* times. The programs they had been admitted to ranged from inpatient residential treatment to outpatient programs. These programs are located within the Detroit Metro area, in rural parts of Michigan, as well as in other states.

The context of treatment and recovery is an informative prism into women's lives. A woman's social vulnerability is magnified through seeking treatment and being a recovering female addict. The combined issues of children, partners, families, as well as financial stability, all play a role in the success of recovery. There were many things I discovered while interviewing women about treatment programs. For example, from listening to some of them and through observation, I found that while in treatment they were often unable to escape from the gendered conditions of their street life. Specifically, the web of gender norms that sometimes involve survival sex and physical abuse does not always abate during treatment. Counselors (and sometimes male users) reproduce some of these norms in the recovery process (see Friedman and Alicea 2001). Furthermore, after they leave treatment, many female users are not prepared to provide financially for themselves or their children.

About midway into this study I divided the women whom I was interviewing into three groups: (1) those who were actively using crack cocaine and participating in street-level sex work; (2) those in the early stages of recovery, and (3) women in recovery three or more years. Throughout the course of the research it was very difficult to keep women from switching categories. There were several occasions when I interviewed a woman who was seemingly making sufficient progress in treatment, and then I would see her months later on the street during my FIT van shift. Even the women who I thought were out of the "danger zone" of initial recovery (two or more years) often slipped back into the "active" category of my sample. There was some movement in the other direction, too. Watching them relapse after several months and years of their sustained effort was more painful than almost any other aspect of the fieldwork process.

HIV/AIDS

When I began this research in the early 1990s, I knew something of the HIV/AIDS virus and HIV/AIDS issues primarily as an informed citizen. However, I was not aware of the important role this virus would play in the lives of my respondents. For instance, when they discovered they were HIV-positive in a demeaning way their reactions were terror, shock, and disavowal. Sometimes I would initially interview a woman and then see her months, or years, later, after she had acquired the HIV/AIDS virus.

As I watched some newly diagnosed women struggle with the implications of HIV/AIDS, I also met others more established within the HIV/AIDS community in Detroit. Over time, I encountered some who were in recovery for three years or longer and they told me about their activities helping others who were HIV-positive. My interest in the variety of their activities grew, and I asked if I could interview them. I made sure that they still fit within my original guidelines: a background of crack use and experience with sex work. I learned from them about the climate for women and HIV/AIDS in the Detroit metropolitan area and the state of Michigan in general.

As they told me how they learned they were HIV-positive and about the journey they had embarked on since then, their narratives led me to consider the relationships between gender, political activism, and stigmatized women.[11] It was through my conversations with these women that my training as a political scientist was stretched taut. Previously, I had been focused on lawbreaking, so the concept of participation and activism for this population—former users/sex workers—seemed remote. Yet the longer I attended their meetings, rallies, and marches, the more it became clear they had organized, mobilized, and participated in their locales in a variety of ways. I became familiar with a growing community of women who were making a difference in Detroit. Besides interviewing them, I also made it a habit to drop by the Partnership and Participation in Health Organization,[12] where a respondent was running one of the largest support groups for women with HIV/AIDS in Detroit. I often was able to visit in an office and be unobtrusive. This allowed me to see the day-to-day challenges of providing services to the HIV community and how respondents negotiated their community work. I put the rest of my energies into understanding this much smaller group of women—a deep sample.

This use of a deep sample is also an approach known as "theoretical sampling" (Glaser and Strauss 1967). Theoretical sampling ensures a type of "representativeness" by allowing a researcher to select informants who have a wide range of the behaviors under study, thereby focusing attention on broad theoretical categories and the meanings that emerge from them.

A central and defining question became, How could I explain and understand the ways in which women politically participated? It was through my own attempt to deeply embed my work in the sixteen women's lives that I was able to see my study come full circle.

THE DEEP SAMPLE'S REPRESENTATIVENESS

The deep sample of women comprises women who were chosen because of their HIV-positive status. Although there were others who were tested for HIV while I had interviewed them, the women of the deep sample were confirmed to be HIV-positive. This cohort, I believe, represent a good cross-section of all the women I interviewed who have histories using crack cocaine and street-level sex work in Detroit. First of all, the deep sample all shared features of the two defining common denominators for choosing women in the overall sample—moderate to heavy crack cocaine use and sex work. These two factors help to differentiate both the deep sample and the overall sample from other women substance users in Detroit who primarily use heroin, pills or other illicit substances, and alcohol.

Given the way the informal drug economies are structured, it would be impossible to obtain a completely random sample of all female crack cocaine–using sex workers. Additionally, it would also not be feasible to obtain a random sample of cocaine using sex workers who were HIV-positive. In terms of the deep sample's pattern of cyclical drug usage and similarity of experiences, I am confident these respondents do not dramatically differ from the overall sample in terms of their educational status, drug use, marital status, or parenting status. Their only true distinction from their counterparts in the overall sample is their HIV-positive status and later interest and participation in their communities.

HOW THE DATA WERE COLLECTED

The initial interviews with all the women were minimally one hour and occasionally an hour and a half long, depending on the circumstances under which I was operating. For the women who constitute the deep sample, I conducted two- to four-hour interviews; these most resemble oral histories. In addition, I became deeply involved in these women's lives, attending support groups, committee meetings, political events, and the various community projects that demanded their time. Informal discussions often took place after heated meetings. During these times, I was there as a researcher and sometimes as a resource person.[13]

The ethnic background of respondents in the entire study sample includes six European Americans, forty-eight African Americans, one Arab American, three Mexican Americans, one Native American, and two Puerto Rican Americans. The majority of respondents are women of color.

Women were financially compensated ten dollars for an hour interview, fifteen dollars for an hour and a half interview, and twenty dollars for a two-hour or longer session. I thought that financially compensating them was of significant importance—especially for the women on the street. Time was definitely equated with money or a score of drugs or both. Financial recompense suggests to an individual that she has important knowledge or skills to impart to the interviewer. It also confers dignity and respect to the interviewee during the interview exchange (Spradley 1979). When I could, I would buy lunches, offer bus and cab fare or a car ride, and provide other minimal monetary support. I did not feel that these activities were out of research bounds, and they also broadly fell within the limits of my grant money (allocated by the university).

If I had not offered money to the respondents, I still believe that the majority of them would have agreed to be interviewed. Why? Because the interview, though not an essentially utopian or therapeutic experience by any means, allowed most of the women to recall and reflect on important, significant experiences in their lives. A prime motivation for many, both those actively using drugs and those with the HIV/AIDS virus, was to correct the public record. The drug using women and women in recovery were very concerned that everyday people or people "not in the life" (of illicit activities) understand the unique challenges in their lives, as different and distinct from the media-created stories and portrayals about women on the street (especially movies like *Boyz N the Hood* and *New Jack City*).

The HIV-positive women wanted to share with me narratives about their ability to triumph over difficult circumstances and were very proud of their accomplishments. Their stories, they felt, were a testimony to survival and resiliency.

People have complex reasons for deciding to be interviewed (Spradley 1979). There were women, on numerous occasions, who turned me down. Additionally, many women of color, particularly African American women, stated they would not have necessarily talked about their experiences with a white researcher.

Fieldnotes that described and analyzed daily events in the lives of the participants were written over the duration of the research period. The final data set consisted of approximately fifteen hundred pages of transcribed interviews,[14] several hundred pages of typed fieldnotes, and a field journal. The bulk of materials were entered into a qualitative software program called NUDIST (Non-Numerical Unstructured Data Indexing Searching and Theorizing). In addition, poems, letters, and copies of announcements or press clippings provided by individual women are part of the final data set. I logged over 216 hours in the field.

Sexuality, Stigma and Fieldwork

Sexuality, as it intersected with stigma, was a dominant theme throughout the gathering of data, and often provided the most consistent challenges and negotiation around my identity. One of the constant dilemmas in the field was, Who was I to talk with these women? People who had some interaction with this population posed this question in multiple ways: social workers, bailiffs, lawyers, hospital staff, and substance abuse counselors. I did not belong to any group or subculture in which these women participated—drug user or sex worker among the dominant aspects of identity. Because my initial entry into the field was around sex work and lawbreaking, in preparing for the field I did some self-reflective work; therefore I thought I was prepared for any difficult situation that might arise. This proved to be another naive assumption on my part. I felt stigmatized both within academia and in the field.

Lynn Chancer (1995) addresses the problems of sexuality in relation to sex work and studies involving sexuality in general. Chancer argues that the norms about what is appropriate outside of academia permeate and are reproduced in academia, and has bearing on what subjects are considered legitimate for study.[15] Chancer is concerned primarily about the sexual content of the study of sex work. She does not discuss implications of the permeation of sexuality within fieldwork.

Men and some women who were not primary respondents often suggested that I would learn nothing from these women, mainly because of their previous sex work and drug histories. They invalidated them as "knowers." Many people's ideas about the population of women I studied are informed through negative media images (Douglas 1994).

I could not escape the sexual and sexualized meanings involved in the lives of women who used drugs, prostituted, and had HIV; they were seen by many as hypersexual.[16] Sexuality and its implications haunted, defined, and played a role in how they often saw themselves. Sexuality in this research overwhelmingly intersected with stigma. Body parts, explicit sexual acts, sexual trauma and abuse—all were events to be confronted, talked about, and discussed, even as my project continued to grow beyond the original emphasis on sex work/lawbreaking. Sexuality—commodified, personified and deified—had to be witnessed and digested if I was to evoke meaningful analyses regarding the women I interviewed. Moreover, throughout this research there was talk of female bodies: doing, performing, and sickening. The female body as a concept was experienced through the daily struggles of recovery, the HIV/AIDS virus, experiences of safe sex, sexual pleasure, sexual trauma, and incest; all had to be confronted when I did interviews. These realities sometimes brought up and mirrored conflictual areas of myself because of my own female body. And although I had not experienced the majority of respondents' specific struggles, there was a resonance to many of their issues because of my race and gender.

The outcome of this discussion reflects on larger ethnographic questions, which revolve around writing about respondents after one has left the field. How does a researcher negotiate sexuality and stigma? How does one talk about marginalized women's bodies that are active in "deviant" activities? How do *I* represent *them* without creating an ever-growing voyeuristic consumption of lower-income women's lives, their "deviant" behavior, and without evoking the public spectacle that has marked public consciousness around race, sex, class, and drugs (see Austin 1992a; Maher 1992; Reeves and Campbell 1994; Campbell 2000)?

I do not have an easy answer for these questions. My general strategy in this book is to try to interrupt traditional assumptions about "these" women, and focus on an analysis that includes their perceptions about the experiences they have had. In conducting this research many of my assumptions about them were challenged, and along with my analysis, I hope to pass on as many unsettling questions as I can.

SECTION TWO: WHY DID SHE SAY THAT? CREATING AND ANALYZING ORAL NARRATIVES

> *What emerges and develops through dialogue are issues—the chaotic and problematic process of two humans thinking and communicating. It is this* rich dialogue *that holds ontological priority, not an impoverished* list.
> —Kristina Minister, "A Feminist Frame for the Oral History Interview"

As the subtitle of this section suggests, I argue that one creates oral narratives from people's "raw" data. I have shaped, studied, and coaxed meanings from the data. It has my stamp of authorship on it. What I have collected over the past few years are in the category of oral narratives; they are not technically life stories, they are not solely semistructured interviews, nor are they typical oral histories. They are narratives, sometimes vignettes, or episodes picked over and worked on, sifted through time and awareness, reattuned for precise moments by respondents and myself. I draw on analyses that understand narratives to be a multilayered event (see Richardson 1990). Using this semifluid frame of oral narratives allows me to give closer attention to the ways in which women construct meaning from the everyday events of their lives, and to highlight the constructed performance aspects of the interview process.

The analysis of the oral narratives has been guided by a framework informed with the concept of feminist methods or principles of inquiry, and particularly multidisciplinary feminist analysis of women's narratives, including autobiographies, biographies, life histories, oral histories, life stories, and testimonies. The diversity of this avenue of research is broad (see generally Behar 1993; Passerini 1987; Gluck and Patai 1991; Naples 2003). Specifically, feminist interventions and innovations within oral history have substantially opened up the field of inquiry. At the beginning of the twenty-first century, there is a heightened attention to how particularly subordinate groups who have been silenced make meaning and understand their lives. Through the use of multiple methods, and especially those that chart and define a life course, researchers highlight intersubjective meanings, which in turn help to reconstruct what we know of human history and the human world. So, from the process of utilizing broad methodological avenues, I was left with the creative richness of oral narratives.

Interviewing

Transforming the interviewing process by paying attention to the gendered context of language—or how women talk—and the diversity of their speech has been one of the major contributions of researchers. Understanding the complexity of how social structures influence women's use of language has been a long and difficult road. Early researchers' aims of just letting women "talk" uninterrupted were in direct contrast to understanding the gendered context of women's speech and socialization (see Devault 1990). Women often express their thoughts in a muted way, tending to frame their concerns through other people's eyes (Anderson and Jack 1991; Devault 1990).

Therefore, as Devault argues, acquiring "useful accounts of women's experiences is not simply a matter of encouraging women to talk" (1990, 99). Contemporary research stresses that when interviewing female subjects, a researcher should go beyond the familiar speech exchanges because of the dominance of ingrained linguistic styles (Devault 1990, 100; Gluck and Patai 1991). Women respondents either tend to think their speech is not interesting or try to conform to an interviewer's expectations. There are two experiences that are common: subjects either talk about others, as opposed to themselves or they question whether their lives constitute an interesting subject. This means a researcher also has trouble when moving outside the expectations of the typical interview format. Others have suggested that "talk" between two women (between researcher and researched) is not necessarily liberating because of the powerlessness of some women, especially vis-à-vis the researcher.

I realized early on that many of the women I would interview were worried about meeting my expectations. My experiences included some individuals who would begin tentatively and be unsure about how to proceed; they often suggested that I would be bored with what they had to say. When they began to talk freely about themselves they frequently stopped and said, "This isn't what you want to hear? Is it?" In her research on gender and the construction of housework, Devault notes a similar situation: "in fact my respondents were uncomfortable because our talk didn't seem like an interview: several stopped in mid-sentence to ask, "Is this really what you want?" (Devault 1990, 99). Devault notes how often women were prepared to self-censor and translate their experiences into those they expected a researcher would want to hear.

I did not consider the process of examining my materials at first as conducting and creating oral narratives—I thought that I was "doing interviews."

This was a technique over which I had some control and a certain amount of skill. It was safe. Throughout many of the early interviews I was focused on facts, details, and events as opposed to understanding the intersubjective cast women brought to making sense of their experiences.

Therefore, early on I focused on their activities involving the use of drugs. Often we probe for "facts" about marginal women who use drugs: How many rocks did you smoke? How many blow jobs did you perform? How often did you go to the crack house? How frequently did you perform safe sex? Initially, I asked these types of questions, which reflected the dominant perceptions of women who used drugs. This was a primary approach to understanding women who smoked cocaine during the early 1990s.[17]

Part of the rationale for the emphasis on facts is because I think deep down, as novice researchers, we are afraid that we will not "find" anything in "women's talk."[18] When respondents strayed off topics and avoided others, I became frustrated, thinking they were presenting a problem or being difficult. Perhaps my questions lacked precision. Indeed, I thought it was my job as an interviewer to rein in respondents and require adherence to an interview schedule. They did not talk about things as *I* wanted them to. I began to ask myself: Why had I undertaken this project if I engaged it by imposing my own worldview on their way of expressing themselves as they discussed their lives?

A shift in the way I began to conduct and think of the materials I was collecting came when I switched from fact gathering to asking what Anderson and Jack suggest is a pivotal question. This is a defining moment for an interviewer engaged in interpretative work: "Is the narrator asked what meanings she makes of her experiences?" (Anderson and Jack 1991, 11). Being engaged in fact finding was helpful and accomplished other necessary goals of the research, but I also became aware of moments when I needed to venture more deeply into a "woman's complex web of relationships and feelings," which meant being patient, following up on silences, and also asking them to make sense of what they were telling me (Anderson and Jack 1991, 13). To consider and to continue to view my subjects as a source of knowledge, I had to step out of the dominant paradigm of interviewing.

The work, then, is to move "methodologically [from] information gathering, where the focus is on the right questions, to interaction, where the focus is on process, on the dynamic unfolding of the subject's viewpoint" (Anderson and Jack 1991, 23). As these authors suggest, traditional interview techniques will prevail until "we can figure out how to release the brakes that these boundaries place on both hearing and memory, our oral histories are likely to confirm the prevailing ideology of women's lives and rob them of their honest voices" (Anderson and Jack 1991, 16–17).[19]

So an attention to the process of how women speak is as important as the subject of their discourse. Thus, this process included mining the data that resembled traditional "woman's talk" as well as looking at interview documents as socially constructed.

Analysis

Anderson and Jack contend that in order analyze women's narratives, "we have to learn to listen in stereo, receiving both the dominant and muted channels clearly and tuning into them carefully to understand the relationship between them" (1991, 11). The concept of attuning in relation to women's speech is an accurate indicator of the action required to understand what they say about themselves. Attuning, or paying attention to what women say as well as charting the missing "channels," allows us more navigational skills as researchers.

Through the analysis of women's texts, however, I found that the literature on listening and recording women's stories asks contradictory things of a researcher, as Devault notes: on the one hand it is assumed that as a female researcher, one could "listen as a woman" (Devault 1990, 101). On the other hand there are exhortations that require researchers to be intensely critical of how constructed the category of gender is (Riessman 1987). This has critical implications for interviewing and analysis.

Here is a brief example of the ways in which these views clashed in my research. Devault (1990) discusses the technique "listening like a woman" (according to her, this means being reflective about how one uses language as a female researcher, and drawing on the experience of being a "woman," a person who is often unempowered or discriminated against in many settings). She posits this as a way to try to understand the manner in which women construct their meanings. This phrase undergirds a contradictory and highly problematic set of assumptions. "Woman" is not an easy or constantly stable category of identity (see Butler 1990; Riley 1988; Feinberg 1996; Spivak 1988).[20]

I asked the respondents to tell me about their worst experiences on the street. I assumed that they were going to tell me about rape, violence, sexual assault, and the like. Indeed, my sense of what "listening like a woman" meant being sympathetic and entailed searching for narratives that would fit under the rubric of "violence against women." I eagerly listened for stories about victimization and disempowerment, descriptions that would confirm one aspect of a feminist frame, which has done much to theorize about the nature of violence against women, and prostitution (see generally Barry 1995; Dworkin 1987; Mackinnon 1989). When their responses did not measure up to what I thought they would say, I pressed them further, assuming they were just circumventing the response, to avoid what

I "knew" to be a troubled set of encounters.[21] In retrospect, through my body language and demeanor I am sure I gave them subtle cues about what I thought an appropriate response should be. After a conversational exchange, one woman asked me, slightly flustered, "You mean rape, or something like that?" Caught off guard, I answered, "Yes." Unfortunately, I conveyed the underlying idea—could there be anything else?

What they did tell me about their worst experiences often had little to do with overt sexual violence during prostitution, and was more attributable to the ways in which crack cocaine use had made them easy targets for humiliation by community members, *both* men and women. Additionally, when there was a sexual component to their "worst experiences" narratives, they often highlighted other aspects of degradation, too. Even when I changed the question to: "What was the most violent thing that has happened to you on the street?" this did not necessarily alter their answers. Their descriptions also contravene some "commonsense" feminist understandings of women's lives on the street (see Maher 1997).

The discord of a researcher's preconceived notions versus their differences from informants' experiences is common to most qualitative researchers. Listening and revising categories is a distinctive iterative process. However, I stress this aspect of the research because not only did I make assumptions about a category called "worst experiences for these women," but "listening like a woman" actually prevented my hearing the variation in their experiences of being stigmatized as a drug user and in other areas of their lives. Constructing a way to understand how women make meaning cannot solely rely on trying to "listen like a woman." Age, class, and race inflections crosscut the categories of "woman."

Another useful technique of analyzing women's narratives has been to help them to create names and meanings for many occurrences that have gone unnoticed and unrecognized (Devault 1990). The aim of research analysis "is the recognition that something is unsaid, and the attempt to hear missing parts of the account" (Devault 1990, 104). This is salient to my approach for exploring respondents' activities concerning their community activism.

Women's activities in the public realm have often been ignored because they are not easily definable (Ackelsberg 1988; Bookman and Morgen 1988; Naples 1998). When analyzing the activities of HIV-positive women, I began to explore the concept of blended and overlapping roles, of activist, helper, and advocate. These roles and their characteristics give meaning to the various activities undertaken by the women that might otherwise go unnamed. Working with the women stretched my notion of what activities were defined as "the political," since women did not frame their meanings solely in political terms and often eschewed the realm of official, organized politics. Additionally, some of the work done by women looked like typical "women's work," which often goes unnoticed (see Naples 1991a, 1991b).

Regarding analysis, I have utilized Anderson and Jack's (1991) heuristic frame, "or ways of listening," to analyze how women understand their actions. Their frame for analyzing women's narratives is composed of three components, stemming from an attention to moral language, metastatements, and the logic of the narrative. Examining moral language means looking at the ways in which a woman describes her actions, which alludes to a disjuncture between her thinking and broader socialized categories—like gender or race. Metastatements can often consist of statements that suggest a woman is evaluating her thinking as an outsider as an "onlooker" (Anderson and Jack 1991, 22). I have modified metastatements to include the self-reflective observations during conversation (usually stopping its flow) to remark on common gendered categories or experiences.

Understanding the logic of a narrative is a way to think about the whole of its structure and its recurring themes, as well as the contradictions between them. I find these to be powerful heuristic tools that enabled me to understand the assumptions of the women's sense of gender obligations as they claim a public voice to engage in HIV/AIDS work and other forms of activism.

Representations of Speech

Finally, I discuss the way respondents' speech is represented on the written page, which has been highlighted in qualitative research. Scholars have called attention to the idea that this process, too, has gendered implications (Devault 1990). Researchers make ultimate decisions ranging from editorial to substantive ones about how to reflect a respondent's speech. Devault notes traditional "practice . . . [that] smoothes out respondents' talk is one way that women's words are distorted; it is often a way of discounting and ignoring those parts of women's experience that are not easily expressed" (1990, 107).

What I have chosen to do in this document is include some dialogue that is rambling or wordy. I have cleaned up the respondents' speech only by taking out the "ums" and "you knows," though I emphasize moments of particular relevance, where there was a struggle in formulating and choosing the appropriate words, or avoidance or discomfort with the question(s). At times I have inserted words to clarify an unusual phrase. Body language is also noted if relevant.

Despite these measures, I have not fully captured the rich orality of the women's speech. The significant turn of phrase that grew to be familiar to my ears, even the differences in how people say familiar words, are not easily conveyed on the written page.

LIMITATIONS OF THE STUDY

Although the research presented thoroughly analyzes the group under study, there are certain limitations that are necessary to mention. Several factors are important to understanding what is missing from this study.

First, members of the medical establishment or of social service agencies in Detroit are not represented, in either the theories or data gathered. These people include medical providers, medical staff, human service workers (at treatment programs), counselors, social workers, psychologists, case managers, and the like. Their understandings and expertise gathered from years of working with this population of stigmatized people are not represented. Including their voices would have allowed for a dialogic probing of how they understood some of the women whom they served.

Second, women in Detroit with HIV/AIDS who were not stigmatized are also not represented in this group of women. It would have been useful to query nonstigmatized HIV-positive women's experiences in public and private hospitals and public and private treatment programs. Given the lack of available services to those with HIV/AIDS, I suspect that women who were diagnosed in the mideighties and early nineties would have faced some similar challenges as compared to women of the deep sample. However, specific experiences and ideas about access to medical treatment, counseling, and support services for nonstigmatized HIV-positive women of Detroit are missing.

The number of women in the deep sample is small and self-selecting. It is possible that women in this cohort were at a specific breaking point in their cycle of addiction when they acquired HIV/AIDS, which then served as a catalyst in ways that may not be true for other types of crack-cocaine-using women. These women may have been more primed to be transformed by the HIV/AIDS virus.

Although, the situation for women with HIV/AIDS has been dire nationally, the uniqueness of Detroit also bears some mention in considering the limitations of the study. Detroit has had an HIV/AIDS epidemic, and Michigan has had high rates of HIV/AIDS infections compared to other midwestern states. Detroit was slow to respond to the HIV/AIDS virus. Also, given the extreme isolation and poverty many Detroit residents faced throughout the eighties (Herron 1995), the confluence of crack use and prostitution may look different when compared to the ways in which stigmatized HIV-positive women from other locales and regions have been able to become organized.

Additionally, all of the participants in this sample were healthy and did not possess or develop full-blown AIDS during the time of research. The majority of the women had been living with the HIV/AIDS virus for under a five-year period. It is not clear what the effects of developing AIDS would do to the resiliency of the respondents or their participation. Developing AIDS would definitely strain the women's personal and professional resolves (and resources), and especially the networks they have helped to create and foster.

Many self-reporting methods of data collection in social sciences research raise questions about the validity and reliability of findings. At best, all self-reports deal with the verisimilitudes of memory and recollection. Observation, multiple methods, and triangulation of data points in this research help to compensate for these challenges.

Since the initial excitement regarding the inroads of feminist-inspired methodology, there has been a growing critical discussion of methodological ethics. Theorists have argued that feminist methods often belie questions of power, authority, and accountability in relation to the people who are subjects of the research (see especially Stacey 1991; Patai 1991). The criticisms of feminist methods have ranged from disbelief in the ability to "represent women's lives" to addressing the responsibility of the researcher to protect subjects and address issues of power. Following these criticisms, there has been a movement to work toward more collaborative, participatory, and even activist research design programs (Gluck and Patai 1991).

This book however, is not a collaborative project. Most respondents (especially those not in the deep sample) were not able to see much of the final text of this book or how I shaped their words. The overall population was a transient one that made it very difficult to follow through on any type of joint authorship or collaborative effort.

However, I met with many women of the deep sample formally and informally, and often would reengage them with conversations about the transcripts; this was not just an exercise to see if their perception of events had changed, but to use that conversation as a point to discuss terms, contradictions, shifts in opinion, and so forth. Their thinking changed over time about subjects (as to be expected), and I note that in the text when applicable. They were easy to reengage about the meanings of their actions.

There are no easy markers for a scholar who becomes involved in a research process like the one I have described in this chapter. As Maher notes, "there are no shortcuts to or through women's lives" (1997, 232). Their journey illuminated harsh realities for me as a social observer and researcher. This book is part of that journey that neither I nor the respondents could completely control. Overall, I accept responsibility for disseminating information in a context where people can rebut, challenge, and ask for more clarification about these words.

## CHAPTER FOUR

Narratives of Injustice: Discovery of the HIV/AIDS Virus

The way I was told about my HIV status was almost as traumatizing as the disease itself.

—Cherise, thirty-two

Dignity is the key word in dealing with AIDS. The women who are active in women and HIV/AIDS issues in Detroit had our dignity stripped away through the very process of finding out we were HIV-positive. We began fighting for our dignity the day we found out we were HIV-positive.

—Cynthia, forty

I never thought that I'd get treated the way that I did by medical providers. But, they really didn't see me that day—as a white woman, what they saw was a dirty crack user, a nobody. Being a white woman only protects you so much.

—Shenna, twenty-five

IN CHAPTER ONE, I have argued that the women's experiences surrounding the context of discovery of the HIV/AIDS virus significantly influenced their future political activity. Their comprehension of those events was a precipitating catalyst to self-recovery, self-empowerment, and later political participation. Delineating their perception of the situation in which they now found themselves after learning they were HIV-positive and the consequences of that discovery, is the focus of this chapter.

Moreover, this chapter explores the resulting *narratives of injustice* arising from the manner in which they were informed they had contracted this serious illness. These narratives of injustice stemmed from what respondents perceived as negligent treatment. These are not just accounts of inconvenience, but rather the ways in which the women were ignored, underserved, and neglected. Their treatment and context of discovery reveal the social dynamics of intersectional stigma discussed toward the end of the chapter.

This neglectful treatment ranged from receiving no or very little useful information regarding the HIV/AIDS virus to actual bias and discrimination based on their drug-using status and prior history of sex work. Because of their social location, they were advised of the HIV/AIDS virus in significantly different ways from many others with the disease. Overall, as they described how they learned they were HIV-positive, respondents would agree that the traumatic event left them, as Georgia has often said, "feeling worth less than an animal laying out to die."

For some women a heightened understanding of the relationship between being HIV-positive and other stigmatized identities was quickly intensified, and for others the occasion was the material for later contemplation that enabled connections between previously hidden, ignored, or unfocused aspects of their identity. They reflected on feelings of being slighted, abused, or unfairly treated. Discovery of their HIV-positive status led them to a series of questions: Why were they treated so poorly? Did they deserve this treatment? Why were they blamed for contracting HIV? Was is it because they were women? Why did others suffer the same disrespect?

The narratives of women who have the HIV/AIDS virus resonate clearly in this chapter and set the stage for further discussions about the relationship between their HIV-positive status, intersectional stigma, and political development.

Narratives of Injustice

Respondents with the HIV/AIDS virus were diagnosed from the years of 1986 to 1996, with those from 1986 to 1992 constituting an early wave.[1]

What is the rationale for the nomenclature "narratives of injustice"? There are several reasons to call attention to the way *they* described this process, and the *researcher*'s subsequent construction of a "second-level narrative," here referred to as a narrative of injustice (Borland 1991, 63). One set of reasons concerns the substantive nature of the accounts and the other set of reasons lie in methodological terrain. We will begin with the substantive emphasis on labeling the women's experiences as narratives.

The accounts of events surrounding their HIV status have a beginning, middle, and end. This includes the discovery, its consequences, and what they did because of it, and often appeared in interviews as an already formed, coherent frame. These accounts constituted a well-organized, well-formulated set of concerns, which each woman presented in conversational context. Although some of these excerpts are brief and are offered concisely to promote analytical clarity, the actual flow of the individual narratives is much longer and fuller. Additionally, these accounts afforded respondents a springboard from which to launch other topics related to their present community work.

The linguistic features of their accounts were striking in that there was careful attention to word choice, repetition, and use of descriptive language; the overall aspects of the accounts had the impact of well-prepared speech acts. These stories were not delivered dryly or by rote, but as an engaging account that could, at times in the relating of it, create an emotional response in the respondent. As Borland notes, the event(s) of personal narrative are simultaneously a "meaning-constructing activity" (1991, 63). She argues that this event: "constitutes both a dynamic interaction between the thinking subject and the narrated event (her own life experience) and between the thinking subject and the narrative event" (63).

What is also contended here is that the fluidity of the narratives and their relative coherence suggest that the women had time to reshape these accounts into a valuable organizing frame, serving as a symbolic and meaningful touchstone in their lives. When asked to discuss their interest in the political world in relation to their activities, they began with their HIV/AIDS diagnosis. Why is this important? Theoretically, because the women's narrative could be interpreted as not only evidence of a life-changing event (discovery of HIV/AIDS), but also as constituting an "origin" story of their politicization. This origin story charts the beginning of their journey into political territory. It is often a focal point for other narratives of political work.

I argue that these early experiences now shaped into narratives describe and formulate what it means to be "a woman newly diagnosed," a category of experience that is critical for respondents. These narratives are a major organizing scheme for respondents and they invoke them while working with clients, sometimes in their public talks and definitely among themselves. The experiences they recount constitute a type of initiation, for themselves and others, providing the basis for the sense of community with other stigmatized women (and men) with HIV/AIDS.

The second reason why these narratives of injustice are important is that methodologically they constitute a "saturation" point. Ethnographers and other qualitative researchers use this term to explain a recurring event, theme, cognitive process, or even word that runs through all cases, and because of its usage is recognizable to the researcher as an important event in the lives of respondents (Glaser and Strauss 1967; Richardson 1990). Saturation points in data signal to the researcher a feeling of epiphany, in that they know that the information they are receiving is of such quality they recognize it immediately in their schema. The women *all* recount how they were cavalierly initially told about their status. That *all* of the women mentioned this attitude toward them, which rested on negligent treatment, when discussing how they later got involved in politics is methodologically significant.

Let us now focus on the injustice component that refers to the women's sense of betrayal, and vulnerability as a consequence. The poor treatment constituted an explosion in their world, almost as severe as learning of the disease. Sometimes they used the words "unjust" and "inhumane" to describe their overall treatment. This schema conveys not only what they felt *at that time*, but also resonates to the larger framework that the women employ *now*. Working for justice on behalf of people with HIV constitutes this larger framework, encompassing both past and present perceptions of the event.

The situations women faced and discussed repeatedly in their accounts about their discovery of the HIV/AIDS virus can be divided into three main themes, which comprise the narrative. These themes demonstrate why this experience traumatized them, and taken together in the context of the overall narrative, they constitute the rubric of injustice.

Respondents were tested for the HIV/AIDS virus in one of five types of place: The Detroit Department of Health, a free neighborhood health clinic, a substance abuse treatment center, prison, or a public hospital.

Theme One: Information About HIV/AIDS, Staff Responsibility, and Staff Follow-up

Several elements comprise theme one. The first is the lack of information, misinformation, or no information within the context of discovery of the HIV/AIDS virus. Respondents were given little or sometimes no information regarding the disease and their condition. Furthermore, they observed that the materials they received seemed inappropriate to their life situation as drug users and as women. This is particularly salient for the women who constitute the early wave of women with the HIV/AIDS virus. Homelessness, drug use, poverty, and abusive partners complicated their lives. Medical and other providers discussed none of these other axes of experience. Later, the women would come to see this as a specific problem concerning the diagnosis and integral support of women with the HIV/AIDS virus.

Other themes related to the lack of information included the unprofessional behavior of the staff in telling a client that she was HIV-positive. In the late eighties and early nineties, facilities like hospitals, clinics, and health departments often did not have a standard procedure for delegating responsibility for informing patients that they were HIV-positive. The HIV/AIDS testing service did not have distinct pre- and posttesting procedures, with counselors for each event, as is now the case in the fairly standard procedure in this country. Such arrangements assure a consistent level of service and support for clients.

Therefore, until recently, anyone in a testing facility could disclose a person's HIV/AIDS status. Respondents often did not know whom to question further about their status. A physician might have been present for the original testing, but ultimately a nurse practitioner or aide informed the patient that she was HIV-positive. The respondent could be left with a nurse, intern, aide, or staff person, or even in one case, a secretary, who might be unaware of the details of the case. For women tested in substance abuse clinics, there often was not a medical professional available.

Another related component of this theme is the lack of follow-up support by professional staff. Women often did not receive any monitoring support for their HIV status. Several respondents mentioned that they were promised medical support and treatment that was never administered.

Theme Two: Focus on Death

The second category of themes, which is found in almost all of the narratives, is the extreme focus, usually by medical providers, on the inevitability of death. Respondents consistently described that after learning of their HIV-positive status, they were, in essence, told to go home and prepare to die. In retrospect, during the early wave of the HIV/AIDS virus, there was not much known about how to cope with the virus; people with HIV were often expected to develop full-blown AIDS and die as a consequence. Respondents said they would have liked information on how to live with the virus, but medical providers offered little of use to them.

Theme Three: Biased Treatment Because of Drug Use

The third and final theme that makes up the narratives of injustice is biased treatment on the part of providers on the basis of confirmed or perceived drug use by the women of the deep sample. Several respondents were tested for HIV/AIDS in relation to some other medical condition (e.g., pregnancy and childbirth). When they went in for an HIV/AIDS test and when information surfaced that the respondents were potential substance users, they were treated differently. As shall soon be demonstrated, comments were made that resulted in them feeling stigmatized. Sometimes respondents said that even if their drug-using status was not known, they believed they received biased treatment from providers because drug use was assumed.

The main themes in these narratives are divided here for purposes of analytical clarity. The experiences in discovery of the HIV/AIDS virus were complex, and often contained at least two of the aforementioned themes embedded in it.

Theme One

Julianna begins this discussion of the first theme. Her narrative is organized around the first theme and its subsidiary elements. She was diagnosed as HIV-positive in 1990.

JULIANNA: *I was going to this one over here [to a treatment program], no actually, I wasn't going to any yet. I wasn't going to any [treatment program] yet. And this commercial comes on TV: Get high, get stupid, get AIDS. Every time it came on, I just looked at it.*

And there the health department's not far from my house. And one day, I just got up and walked over. I said, you know, I got high, I sure am stupid [laughter from both interviewer and interviewee]. *And I just had to know. And so I went around there to get the test. And when I came back it was positive.*[2] *And then they muffed it up. They muffed up telling me—They muffed that all up, one person thought the other person had told me and they didn't. So you know, that was really messed up. Let me explain.*

. . . I went in, and the aide sent me to a nurse, and then that nurse sent me back to the first lady, and I went back to the first lady, and she just launched this spiel, and started handing me these pamphlets. I said, so I guess you're telling me I'm positive.

"Oh, she didn't tell you?" [the aide asked]. *Oh, no, gang slap her. So I found out I was positive. First thing ran across my head was my baby's going to die.[3] That's the first thing I thought about.*

I'm like, well I'm positive, that means she's positive. So, I spent the next three years getting her into the hospital and making sure everything, she was taken care of.

They just handed me that mess [pamphlets] *and told me to get ready to die,[4] you know, I really didn't have much to hope for.*

I had a friend, a social worker, who I had been talking to over the years. She was there when I got tested. And if it wasn't for her [being there], I probably would have gang slapped them. Because I almost dropped my baby. I almost dropped her.

Their bedside manner was nil. They were totally unprofessional about this. I'm like, this is not the way [you tell people], you know. You knew I was coming back. You knew I was coming back.

There weren't on-site counselors in 1990. All this stuff just came into being in the last few years, because we fought for it. There were no rules then. The nurse told you. The social worker might tell you. It was real confusing. It wasn't someone's set responsibility. It's unbelievable.

Now you have pre- and posttest counselors. They didn't have that then. They didn't have any of that. And there are [now] set people whose responsibility it is to inform people of their status. So, yeah, that was a poor, poor experience. Especially coming from the health department. Supposedly the powers that be [delivered strongly].

Valerie was attacked and raped in her home by a stranger and was not a heavy crack cocaine user at the time. She was diagnosed in Parker Hospital in 1991.[5]

VALERIE: *I called the police. He [the attacker] told me not to, but afterwards, I called my friend, and he's like, "You got to call the police, you got to call the police." I went to Parker, and did all this stuff, but I didn't ask for a test right away. So then, in March, I had my baby. In March, I had my baby. And I tested, and I was positive.*

I hate Parker Hospital. I hope you're not with them [interviewer assures her that she is not affiliated with Parker Hospital]. *Because they did the HIV/AIDS pretest and I went back there, and it was time for me to go home. I'm dressed, my baby's dressed, my mamma's there, ready to go.*

The doctor kept coming in and out, and she finally stopped me at the door and said, "I'm sorry, you're [HIV] positive." And that was the extent of my counseling. So there I was, going out the door—

MICHELE: *That's it?*

VALERIE: *Out the door.*
MICHELE: *That's amazing.*
VALERIE: *Not a damn thing.*

We continue with Daria, who was introduced in an earlier chapter. She found out her HIV-positive status through her experiences in prison in 1991. She was serving a sentence for petty larceny:

> DARIA: *I found out I was HIV-positive through the penitentiary system. This was in December 1991.*
> MICHELE: *How did you feel?*
> DARIA: *Well, at the time I didn't feel nothing. I was just told that I had HIV, and I needed to quit smoking cigarettes. Totally nothing. It hadn't come nationwide. I really think they didn't start putting it in the papers and on TV until about 1994. So it was still like, no one really knew. So after I got out of prison, I had nobody—nobody didn't never bring it up to my attention again, so I never talked about it anymore.*
>   *And I went on with my life. But inside I was really angry. I wouldn't know how angry until later. I didn't even think about how ignorant I was in prison until later. I was so ignorant about what I needed to do for myself. That ignorance, mine and theirs, cost me years off my life.*

What is striking about Daria's comments is that in 1991 *there were* national health campaigns about the severity of the HIV/AIDS virus. Detroit and the state of Michigan had been slow in responding to the HIV/AIDS crisis, however, as compared to other large cities. Given that many of the women did not think of themselves at risk for the disease, along with the fact that raising local awareness about HIV/AIDS was slow, presents other reasons for the relative lack of information regarding the HIV/AIDS virus.

Georgia also discovered she was HIV-positive in prison in 1995. She originally requested to see a doctor for another problem and had been asked to take an HIV/AIDS test, to which she consented.

> GEORGIA: *Let me tell you, when I found out I had the virus—that was the worst day of my life. They called me in, the head correctional officer, and some other people who worked there called me into the office, and quizzed me, you know what I'm saying? Asked me how I was doing, and that kind of small chitchat shit. And then they told me that I had HIV. And it was really shocking to me, because that December, I went to Hope for Us[6] to be tested for HIV, OK? It was three men and one woman who was in the office, by the way, so I was doubly embarrassed. I did not want those male guards to know anything about me.*
> MICHELE: *Did they [the prison staff] offer you support?*

GEORGIA: *Support? They told me they would, but they never did. They didn't even have books in the prison library on HIV or anything. You know. I'm trying to sue them now, because for a long time I had [undiagnosed] second-degree syphilis. Earlier I had asked to see a doctor. That was the original reason I wanted to go to the doctor, then I get called in, and found out I had HIV. I kept feeling something strange. I had a strange odor [points to her groin]. But I had syphilis because I broke out with bumps all over, you know what I'm saying?*

And I kept begging them and begging them to give me antibiotics, or run an STD [test] on me. I said "You see that I got HIV, check me for other things." But they didn't check me out or anything for a long long time. They let me go on like that.

They had a male support group for HIV, if I wanted to go to that. They hadn't established a women's one yet. And the thing about it, I asked to see the psychiatrist and he put me on a waiting list, and I wait and wait. You know. You know what I'm saying? It was like awful.

MICHELE: *How did you feel?*

GEORGIA: *Oh, scared to death, you know what I'm saying? It hurt more, me being really scared. I couldn't think, because I was so scared.*

As soon as I come out from prison, between the tears, I went straight to find a good doctor, someone who could help me. It was really hard for me to find a place though to talk about HIV. I'd have taken anything, scraps, I'd have taken those. They still only had services for men at most places I checked . . . and that was just a few years ago. It's like the women were tucked away somewhere, and I didn't know how to find them. So many programs really don't offer none of what women need, and this is why I want to get into HIV work.

That day we spoke, she was applying for a state grant that helps women with the HIV/AIDS virus attend special classes and conferences.[7]

Simone was tested through a counseling program in an outpatient drug treatment center in 1990.

SIMONE: *They was very, very ugly with it [the people who told her she was HIV positive]. OK. I always went there for ulcers on my legs [for previous heroin use], so that gave them the reason to want to question whether I had the virus or not. So they asked me, they did ask me if I wanted to take a test, and I agreed. I had to sign the papers. I wasn't counseled before or after. I was going through so many things back then, but the test results came in, they told me I had the virus. They said, "You have HIV. You have something called AIDS."*

They didn't give me no referrals, they didn't give me no counseling before or after or anything. They didn't refer me to a doctor or anything.

We will return to Simone's understanding of that time later in the chapter. Now we turn to Anna. Anna was diagnosed at Parker Hospital (the same hospital Valerie went to). She was someone who regularly chose to get tested for the HIV/AIDS virus.

ANNA: *I used to go to Hispanic Community Support (HCS),*[8] *and I always got tested. And then when I met this guy that I'm living with, I told him one night. I said, "You know, we need to go and find out about HIV. I want to get tested."*

I had been out on the streets off and on for years, and I had heard that HIV was some God deadly stuff. So I went to the hospital where I could get free testing.

I come back, and I had to wait forever, and the nurse was the one who told me. She looked me up and down and said, "Anna you have HIV. Do you know what that really is?"

I broke down in tears, my face was red and everything . . . tears, tears . . . and the nurse looked like she was upset at me. She gave me some things to read, and said that I would get a follow-up call. And that was it. I never heard nothing from them . . . and I waited by that phone, for once I even stayed off the street.

Anna said there was not a follow-up call or any other type of support services. Some of the respondents said they never got a promised follow-up call from a doctor or health official.

Two of the women interviewed said they were offered a bit more information and counseling than only pamphlets. Robin took an opportunity to go to treatment when it was offered, soon after her test, and Charlene said she refused initial help at first. Despite this, however, both Robin and Charlene thought that the overall service surrounding HIV/AIDS information, intervention, and treatment they received was inadequate and substandard. What is striking about all of their narratives about acquiring the HIV/AIDS virus is the *consistency* with which they described their poor treatment, and that they later characterized these events as traumatic and life changing.

Theme Two

The second major theme of the women's narratives is that of the concentration by medical providers and human service workers on the inevitability of death of the women diagnosed with the HIV/AIDS virus. Respondents discussed at length the type of negative effect it had on them; those women who do public speaking constantly stress ways of living, not dying, with the disease.

The Detroit Health Department in early 1994 diagnosed Shelly with HIV. She was also not given any counseling. She stressed repeatedly in the interview that the doctors and nurses acted as if she was "going to die immediately." During her telling of the narrative, she often became upset, even when she spoke about her experiences in public. She discussed her immediate response to the news:

SHELLY: *They just told me, the lady, she told me I had it. And she said, "You got HIV, and you're going to die one day."*

. . . Yep. They introduced me to this doctor, and he took me over to Dr. Riley. So when I talked to her, I was on this focus of dying thing, you know. And she said, "Well,

you ain't going to die tomorrow . . . it might be six months, it might be a year." Six months to a year?! So I'm really panicking now. You know, they ain't never tell me that I might be around for a while. All they kept saying, "It can happen at any time." So I walked around with this fear. . . . Just scared senseless. I was just freaked out. And I figured as I'm going to sleep, I might not wake up like my sister. You know, because my sister died in her sleep. I said, "I'm going to die in my sleep." So I was going through an emotional void. I was just freaked out [all delivered very excitedly].
MICHELE: *Was any counseling offered to you?*
SHELLY: *No, nothing.*[9]

Kitt was diagnosed with the HIV/AIDS virus during late 1995 in a public hospital. She went for the test after a suggestion by a psychiatrist.

KITT: *They asked me whether I had kids and I replied, "No."*

The doctor nodded. "Well, that will make it a lot more easier on you when you die. It's so much harder when people have families. They have many demands on their time."

Die? [waves hands frantically in front of face]. *Oh, I wanted to scream. I didn't in no way want to hear about death, my death, and that's all he talked about the whole time I was there, preparing me for death.*

I couldn't. I didn't know what to say. It's like if I could've opened my mouth, I would've screamed at him for everything that had happened to me at that point in my life, on top of what he was telling me.

Respondents recounted that there was a constant stress on death, possibly immediate, and no doubt inevitable. Little to no hope was given to women that they might be able to live with this disease. As their discussion indicates, the medical providers were either inept at explaining what possibilities lay ahead for the women or they did not believe it possible for the women to live a full life with what they knew medically about the virus. Either way, this focus on death contributed to making the women feel entirely hopeless and triggered a desperate set of responses.

Theme Three

The last and final theme to be considered in this aspect of women's narratives is the perception of biased treatment. Because of their drug-using status, many respondents were already wary of accessing public facilities like hospitals, due to prior negative experiences. For a typical substance abuser, the hospital, in particular, is not a place of sanctuary.

Nicole was the only woman among the sixteen to lose a child because of perinatal transmission of the HIV/AIDS virus. This event, along with her experience of discovering she was infected, helped her to later confront issues of women with HIV; she empathizes with pregnant women who have HIV, and has devoted much of her time to this population.

NICOLE: *I was still using, and I was pregnant at the time. And these guys that was in my house, they was rolling. The dope was so plentiful then that I didn't even think about stopping to use during my pregnancy. I got high, had unprotected sex, plenty of unprotected sex. I didn't think about a condom, using no protection or anything like that. And once my baby was born, about three weeks later, they called me to come down to the hospital because he was so sick. And then they told me that they had tested my baby, and he was HIV-positive.*

That one day, I was in a state of denial, because I didn't know that it was me that was HIV-positive, I just thought it was my baby. Because I didn't know anything about being HIV. Only thing I heard about HIV and AIDS was that these gay guys was dying from AIDS, so I just thought it was them. But my girlfriend, she went home, and she read about it and she called me up and she said the only way the baby could be HIV-positive was through the mother's blood. And I said, "That can't be true." And she said, "Well, that's what I read." So I went to the doctor and found out it was all true. They were so unhelpful it borders on ridiculous; all the information I received from the doctor couldn't have taken more than ten minutes—and that's for both me and my baby. They already had found traces of crack in my system, so they were pretty rude to me. They talked to me as if I was a child, and just, you know, out of it. They asked me a few questions about my other son, and I felt I had to keep saying, I'm a good mother. I'm a good mother. I felt as if everyone could tell what I had been doing.

Shenna in 1995 went to a public hospital for an HIV/AIDS test and found out she was HIV-positive. She expressed disbelief. She had previously confided in the aide that she used crack cocaine. Shenna discussed the aide's responses:

SHENNA: *As I kept saying, "I don't believe this . . . I don't believe this," this woman who told me my results said: "Well, did you think it was impossible for you to get HIV because you smoke crack? You better think about that before you get back on your pipe." She left me some pamphlets and then left the room.*

Michele, I just broke down in tears. I didn't know what to say. . . . I knew she shouldn't be saying that to me, but what could I say? I never want another woman to go through the experience that I went through, no matter what she did, or who she is.

Billy Jean was diagnosed in 1993:

BILLY JEAN: *Here comes the doctor. The doctor said, "You're pregnant." And he looked at me and I looked at him, and I said, Excuse me you must have made a mistake. I'm not pregnant. And he's scratching his head, he's like, "No, no." I said, Well, can you tell me how far along I am? And he asked me while I was there in the hospital was it a chance that I, was I HIV-positive? And I'm like no! He wanted me to take an HIV/AIDS test. I felt pressured to take the test.*

. . . From the [earlier] blood work, he said they had already found traces of crack cocaine in my system. I got really scared. It was my first baby, you know and I was worried that if I didn't take the test, they'd call protective services, or something. Like now I know they can't do that, but I sure didn't know that then. So I let them take the test. Well, then he consulted with another doctor and they transferred me to Brightline Hospital[10] because they have the high-risk pregnancy clinic called Care for You.[11] I had to retake the test there. As I'm leaving, the doctors done left in a huff and the nurse is giving me more forms to fill out and she says,

"Give your baby a better chance than you've given yourself. Don't let it get addicted to drugs." And let me tell you, she didn't say it none too friendly.

Yeah, so anyway I go to Care for You. They did a two-week HIV test thing, but they called me back in less than a week. Called my sister's house, called my daddy's house. And I knew, I had a funny feeling that they were going to tell me that I was HIV-positive. But I went on and heard what she had to say because I was concerned because I was carrying a baby. And that's the only reason why I took the test. Other than that, I would have never took the test. I'm glad I did in the end, because my baby's healthy now. And once they told me, I was devastated.

The doctor told me, "We found traces of crack cocaine in your system, and you're HIV-positive. We can't do nothing for you, here." And, I mean she said it so terrible. So mean. I can't even describe how she really said it to me. And here is it was supposed to be a clinic for women with problems [sucks her teeth]. They didn't have any facilities for women like me who was pregnant and had HIV.

After the doctor left, some other lady there told me I had to get out of the room, because they was waiting on other patients. They didn't offer no kind of support or nothing.[12]

Constance had not been feeling well for a long while during her crack use. She was tested at a public hospital in 1994.

CONSTANCE: *With me having been a nurse I immediately was teed off at the service I was getting. When I went back to get my information, after the pretest, you know, I asked to see a doctor. And they told me only aides perform this part of the test. I could make an appointment if I did find out I was positive to see a doctor, but they didn't specialize in care of HIV/AIDS patients. They also asked me if I used drugs and I said no. I didn't want to volunteer any information I didn't have to and you know what the aide said to me later after he finished telling me I was HIV-positive?*

"Why are you going to lie now? Drugs is a part of the problem."

Representatives of doctors are not supposed to make sharp comments like that. I was so angry I was speechless.

You know he left the room and then I didn't see him again. Another aide came back in to check on me, and asked me if I had someone I could call to pick me up from the hospital. They gave me some diddle squat information about the virus.

Several respondents (e.g., Julianna and Constance) expected to be treated fairly in medical facilities.[13] For others, these experiences confirmed several already negative impressions they had about accessing public institutions, primarily because of their drug-using status. During the period when many women discovered they were HIV-positive, they were in a city and state whose preparations for the HIV/AIDS virus was not as far reaching compared to other regions of the country. We return to Shenna. I was fortunate enough to listen to a talk she gave in 1997 to a community center on the east side of Detroit that had sponsored a panel on women and HIV/AIDS:

I have talked to many women about this disease. I stand here with the wisdom of those women. Our stories are very similar. If you use drugs and happen to be HIV-positive do not expect compassion, support, or sympathy by and large. I was treated poorly and was made to feel like a second-class citizen. Other women have told me similar stories of how they were treated—the looks, the taunts, the wisecracks or remarks that made her cry. We keep trying to educate doctors and staff and train people to not discriminate. How is a woman supposed to feel safe enough to come back and get services if when she is tested and told her results, she is humiliated?

Consequences of the Discovery of the HIV/AIDS Virus

Once they found out they were HIV-positive, the women were in a state of shock, denial, and rage. Having few resources at their disposal and feeling the burden and stigma of being HIV-positive, they felt they could not easily turn to relatives, associates, friends, or even lovers. The fear of their disease and how people would view them was a salient mediating factor in their perception of what their options were.

We return to Shelly's understanding of that experience. During the interview I asked her if she told anyone about her HIV-positive discovery. What she reveals parallels the state of mind (if not the actions) of other respondents:

SHELLY: *Nope. I was scared. I wanted to tell somebody, but I figured people would hurt me.[14] I kept it to myself. And I turned tricks as a prostitute for a few years after I knew I was HIV-positive. I was a prostitute on the streets with—spreading HIV around, until I got tired, and I told the judge to lock me up. That's how I got into my first treatment center. Because they [the judge] told me I was a deadly weapon. I told them how long I had been out there and I was tired. And I just wanted somebody to listen and help me* [emphasis added].

Although Shelly's experience was by far the most dramatic of the respondents, they all recounted a period of heavy drug use, reckless activities, episodes of despair and sometimes attempted suicide.

We also return to Simone. She was interviewed in 1995 about her HIV-status:

That's why I'm mad with this you know, I am, because I wouldn't have just said,
"Fuck it, I'm going out on the street and kill myself with the drugs because I'm going
to die anyway." You know, that's the attitude I had. I had it because I wasn't counseled.
I really did the drugs. There was no one I could talk with. . . . And now, like I said,
I've been going to group and doing my part, . . . They really should have counseled me,
and just not treated me so badly. Should have been someone there before and after.
I didn't really know that then.

Simone was interviewed again in 1996.

I wished I could take that person now and just choke the shit out of him, you know.
Because, I just gave up altogether when they told me that [she was HIV-positive]. I'm
going to die anyway, you know. And I didn't have no one there for support, no nothing.
Nothing. It's a shame. Because women don't have to give up . . . women they just give
up altogether if they aren't given some support, and knowledge. Knowledge is what
counts. They need to know so they don't go drinking and drugging themselves to
death.

Simone and Shelly's testimonies illustrate what other women have confided: the way that they were told about their HIV status and their experience with providers pushed them deeper into isolation and drug using. Also, because of current or former lifestyles, they were very afraid to seek help of any kind. Almost every one of the sixteen women went through a period of intensive drug use after discovering she was HIV-positive, even if she was not a heavy user at the time.

Respondents in interviews repeatedly told me how dissatisfied they were that no one talked to them about substance abuse or the other material conditions of their lives when they were given the test results. For example, Kitt was homeless when she found out she was HIV-positive. She needed and wanted services to deal with her homelessness.

Billy Jean's discussion of her family and partner's reaction communicates an example of the immediate stigmatizing consequences she faced. She was homeless at the time, pregnant, and living between boyfriends and the streets. Soon after learning she was HIV-positive, she came home and told her family.

BILLY JEAN: *My father said to me, "But you can't come back here to live."*
At the same time once the baby's daddy found out, he cried like a baby. He said with
this anger in his voice, "I don't know nothing about it! If it's mine kill it."[15]
. . . But for some reason, he [the baby's father] had a change of heart. Because after
he found out how my family was treating me—they told me I had to leave because
I had the plague—he told me to come on back. And he started to re-educate himself

because of me, because later that year I called the HIV/AIDS hotline to get
information, and that's where it all began for me.

But I used before that. I thought, hey, I'm not going to be on this earth long. I used
while I was pregnant. It was one of my worse periods.

Billy Jean fits other women's descriptions of their families' reaction to
their HIV/AIDS status.

In the last five years women of the deep sample have worked together to
change many of the testing procedures and counseling services for women
newly diagnosed with HIV/AIDS. However, as the fieldnote below suggests,
as late as 1997 some women (in particular drug users) who are tested were
still not treated with respect, nor did they perceive that the agency or institution handled their problems well. The fieldnote also speaks to the level of
stigma that women perceived, and how little it seems certain situations had
changed for women discovering their HIV-positive status in Detroit:

I just stopped by Participation and Partnership in Health Organization
(PPHO) to see how women were doing, and possibly to have lunch with
Nicole.[16] There was a big trip retreat going on, and many women were waiting
for the van outside. I saw people that I knew there, and that was really nice—
like Julianna and Simone whom I had interviewed early on. Simone looked
great, she had a head full of delicious looking, thickly coiled luscious braids.

While waiting outside, I struck up a conversation easily with a woman, newly
diagnosed, who was just getting involved with the support group. I asked her
how she liked it there and she bluntly asked: "You're not scared to be around
us?" And, I immediately thought how remarkable and sad, that someone with
HIV would have to worry whether strangers are going to be uncomfortable or
"scared" around them. And I assured her that "No. I wasn't scared."

She said that she was still asking questions about what the virus meant to her.
She liked this place [PPHO] better than Hope for Us. This tends to corrobo-
rate my early finding that some places have very bad reputations for diagnosing
women with HIV.

And she said that [when they told her she was HIV-positive] they told her to
go home—with no follow-up or nothing. I think that was Hope for Us. The
woman said that at the Participation and Partnership in Health Organization
the women were so sweet and nice.

The conversation turned to economics, which it usually does. The women
were talking about their food stamp allotment which is a pitiful $54 a month.
They intimated to me, "How can you eat healthy on that type of money? You
have to buy cheap foods, chicken backs, and that type of thing, things which
stretch." It made me think of the other consequences of being poor—not being
able to buy good food; especially this is a problem when you are trying to be
healthy and recover from a serious illness. (Fieldnote, March 1997)

INTERSECTIONAL STIGMA AS A CONTRIBUTING FACTOR

Attention to the interrelated relationships between race, class, and gender as expressed through the context of intersectional stigma helps us to more fully comprehend the larger social processes influencing respondents' experiences discovering they were HIV-positive. I argue that they were already vulnerable to receiving negative and inferior treatment regarding their HIV/AIDS status—being primarily women of color, of low-income status, sex workers, and drug users. Additionally, as crack cocaine users their positioning within the informal drug economy of Detroit was highly racialized.[17]

All the women were tested in what could be thought of as primarily public institutions. They belong to a class of people whose primary or only health care access is to public health facilities. Many were tested in public hospitals, public clinics, and publicly funded substance abuse treatment centers. The type of treatment and care a woman receives in these public facilities as compared to the quality of services in private facilities is strikingly different. Publicly funded institutions are not typically the most receptive to lower-income stigmatized women. A private hospital might have dealt with them in a less stigmatizing manner, and offered substance abuse treatment or counseling or both for other problems.[18]

There is also ample research to substantiate that African Americans, in particular, face discrimination from the medical establishment in both gaining access and securing comprehensive treatment (see American Medical Association 2001). It is difficult for such a woman to get the services she needs if she suspects that a provider is discriminating against her during a medical interview. Shelia Battle, an African American medical social worker, suggests that the approach a medical provider takes in dealing with a client "has a very real impact on the success or failure of the relationship they have with one another" (1997, 287).[19]

Gender is also an important explanatory factor in the status of research and knowledge that existed in the late eighties and early nineties in regard to women with HIV. As discussed in chapter 1, it has been a long and slow journey for women with HIV/AIDS to receive any type of attention at all. Women with HIV/AIDS were last on the list to get services. The medical establishment's response throughout the 1980s was a neglectful one, raising other critiques of ignorance and misogyny in relation to female health (see Ehrenreich and English 1973). The overall national lack of context and research on women with HIV/AIDS contributed to their poor treatment during the 1980s and early 1990s (see Patton 1994). From the lack of clinical studies on women's specific physiological responses to HIV and AIDS—to the actual visibility of HIV-positive women, women were made aware of their second-class citizenship (ACT/UP New York Women and AIDS Book Group 1992; Schneider and Stoller 1995). As Stoller notes:

> As late into the epidemic as 1989, women were still invisible to medical and social services as people with AIDS. By 1995, there had been some change, but the struggle was still going on to have women included in the very definition of AIDS by the Centers for Disease Control (CDC). (1998, 11)

The one area of sustained research is on the perinatal treatment of women with HIV; there has been intense societal concern about mothers passing the HIV/AIDS virus on to their children:[20]

> Most medical attention to women in the epidemic has actually been on pregnant women and pediatric AIDS cases. There is virtually nothing known medically about AIDS in nonpregnant women. Until recently, U.S. women have not been included in clinical trials. And many of the opportunistic infections associated with HIV in women, such as invasive cervical cancer and pulmonary tuberculosis, became part of the U.S. Centers for Disease Control "official" definition of AIDS only in 1993. (Schneider and Stoller 1995, 8)

When discussing this situation and wondering about why so many women had similar experiences, I turned to Nicole to elicit her understanding of the context of HIV/AIDS for women. She talked at length about the invisibility of women with HIV/AIDS and the challenges that she faced in working with medical providers on these perplexing problems:

NICOLE: *They [doctors] never did want to recognize women having HIV or AIDS. And right now, some doctors still find it hard to believe that women can be HIV-positive. They won't always test them for HIV. If a lady came in right now with a bad yeast infection—they wouldn't test them for HIV.[21] They wouldn't say, "Well, do you want to take an HIV antibody test or anything like that?" They'll just test them for pneumonia. That's why, a lot of women, some women get sicker quicker. And then, once they do find out she has HIV, there's no guarantee a doctor is going to know where to send her for special services. There's no guarantee they are going to be helpful to her.*

I'm on a committee now, well we're going to be meeting for the next four months, and we already had two meetings. It's a committee on perinatal transmission. I told the doctor that's on it, he's the co-chair, I'm a co-chair, and this lady named Frances is another co-chair. And I told the doctor, I said, "You got your work cut out for you." I said, "Because even though we may bring the doctors in here and train them, they're still not going to be HIV-friendly." You know what I'm saying? It's not going to be that way.

MICHELE: *Can you tell me what HIV-friendly means?*

NICOLE: *Compassionate. You know. Understanding of a mother coming in with her children, you know, that they need to have some doctor's office equipped with a little day care or something. Something to accommodate the mothers that come in. They might need to have an earlier appointment or something. Training staff people to speak with women and do follow-up. A lot of nurses are real snotty. Yeah.*

MICHELE: *Did the doctor on the committee know what you were talking about?*
NICOLE: *Oh, he knew what I was talking about. Yeah, he knew exactly what I was talking about. And when I told him HIV-friendly, he knew exactly what I was talking about. I'm just explaining it to you.*

Another related and interwoven contributing factor is the fact that the women were drug users, of crack cocaine, a drug which is highly stigmatized for women of color and women who live in urban areas (Zerai and Banks 2002; Campbell 2000; Maher 1997). The changes in sentencing laws regarding crack ocaine have contributed to higher numbers of Latina and African American women in prisons and jails (Mauer and Huling 1995). Women, particularly African American women, were punished by the legal system, and often blamed for the drug abuse in communities (Maher 1992). Research examining the differential effects of stigma between male and female users found that women users are more stigmatized than their male counterparts and also receive less parental support (Shayne and Kaplan 1991).

The confluence of race, gender, and substance use is important in this discussion given Billy Jean's experience. Billy Jean was a pregnant, drug-using African American woman. It is interesting to note that she was turned away from a clinic designed to help women with high-risk pregnancies. She was very worried about the possible proceedings that could have taken place against her, as are most of the women from my larger sample who use drugs and have children. Chasnoff's (1990) research on white women and black women pregnant substance users who were tested for drug use in both public clinics and private care is revealing. African American women in this study were nearly ten times more likely to be reported by physicians to the police for substance abuse (Chasnoff 1990), despite the fact that the white women in the study tested positive for drug use during their pregnancy at rates similar to black women.

It is not just that they found out that they were HIV-positive, which made them become interested in HIV/AIDS issues. It was the negative experiences surrounding their discovery, and the later reflection on what might have generated these attitudes that contributed to future political activity. All this suggested to them that they, as women, were viewed differently from men when it came to the HIV/AIDS virus.

For women of the deep sample these events were the catalysts for self and societal examination. They formed a major life turning point. As they talked to one another and reflected on their problems, many of the group concluded that the initial neglect and treatment of their HIV-positive status was a result of being stigmatized women along several axes. Some, on their own or with others, made connections about the multiple areas of inequality they faced. How they dealt with the multiple challenges are the topics of the next two chapters.

## CHAPTER FIVE

Life Reconstruction and the Development of Nontraditional Political Resources

What Is Life Reconstruction?

In the literature on empowerment and women with HIV/AIDS, there has been little research that has sought to document the specific ways women empower themselves, or what types of special processes women with the HIV/AIDS virus might undergo along the way of becoming politicized. Calling this process *life reconstruction* highlights some specific methods and techniques these respondents employed en route to their own and others' empowerment. Life reconstruction also highlights microlevel processes, which constitute for the women a set of tools for a reframing and redirection of the cumulative effects of HIV-stigma. Chapter 6 explores in depth the gendered aspects of the life reconstruction process.

This chapter discusses the concept of life reconstruction as a process integral to the development of political empowerment for the respondents. It specifically focuses on the external resources discovered, cultivated, and used that created the conditions for internal resources to develop. During substance abuse treatment and recovery, for example, respondents were introduced to therapy, spirituality, the language of advocacy, advocacy education, and to city- and state-sponsored programs for HIV-positive women. After being exposed to some of the rudiments of advocacy, respondents adapted, expanded, and improved upon this foundation as they became active in their communities.

As the recovery and gender identity components of life reconstruction are highly relational and interactive categories, both spheres have consequences for respondents' ability to stay drug-free.

Life reconstruction although broken apart for analytic clarity, comprised a set of ongoing activities. Each of the women took a specific path in the life reconstruction process, yet the end result was one of commonality and shared experiences. I argue that the degree to which respondents were able to maintain their later participation depended on how much they gained from this process. Those who have not been able to successfully undergo this process are hindered in the development of a "public voice." A public voice is a term I use to describe the outcome of acceptance and responsibility about being a woman with HIV/AIDS. I argue the development of a public voice facilitates other modes of participation.

Life reconstruction is not a perfect, complete, nor linear process. Women periodically relapsed with drugs. There were times they actively struggled with the older, ingrained negative definitions about being HIV-positive, and with their newer concepts of "what it means to be a woman with HIV/AIDS." Throughout the process, the women ranged widely as to the degree that they were able to actively embrace, support, and respect themselves, or one another. At various points over the course of this research women fared better with some aspects of the process than others. Those who were able to maintain their political activities were women who consistently struggled through all of the specific processes outlined.

THE ROLE OF RESOURCES

The question of resources as necessary to political life is a reccurring theme in understanding the nature of political participation. Resources have been identified as materials, skills and abilities that help facilitate access to political participation, and even provide transferable skills that can be utilized in other areas. Resources that are broadly well documented include time, money, and civic skills (see Rosenstone and Hansen 1993; Schlozman, Burns, and Verba 1994). Resources in this research are thought of as constituting a continuum of external and internal resources that bring both tangible and intangible benefits partially derived from the treatment process. For this group their remarkable ability to become and stay politically active stems from almost none of the traditional features of resources that have been central to theorizing about participation.

The data made it necessary to confront the inadequacies of understanding HIV-positive women's experiences in treatment. So although they felt stigmatized, and often might have been the only HIV positive women in a group—they were still able to "mine" the program and work on issues that were directly helpful to them. The concept of resources helps make visible individual efforts at recovery in these contexts; it also enables us to identify what before has gone unnoticed.

This work extends the study of Boehmer (2000) on a comparison between breast cancer activism and HIV/AIDS activism by women. She argues that the survival skills that comprise the HIV activism are rooted in an outsider and marginal culture:

> They [survival skills] stem from belonging to a counterculture or subculture that has forced its members to develop skills of survival and resistance from a seemingly powerless place. Boehmer 2000 (46)

Boehmer does not elaborate on the varied nature of these "skills" for the HIV/AIDS activists or provide an extensive discussion of what constitutes survival skills. Resources go beyond the idea of survival skills for explaining my respondents' paths to activism. Although it is true that they use their experiential knowledge as components of their activism, I argue that to make visible the full and dynamic spectrum of the ways that women participate, we must acknowledge the full palette of local aptitudes, competencies, and talents that women utilized. My emphasis remains on calling the full spectrum that I witnessed as resources in the broadest sense. By doing so it suggests that the mechanisms of empowerment are not just reducible to "life aptitudes" but are part of a varied and interactive web of identifiable steps and processes. Respondents did not have an innate or inherent sense of how to deal with being stigmatized. Through the process of observation, reflection, dialogue, and resistance they were able to confront the indices of stigma. This work demonstrates the possibility that a person can develop internal and utilize external resources despite ongoing stigmatization.

These resources, although context specific, may help other researchers capture aspects of the implicit dynamics that have politicized women's experiences with HIV/AIDS. This focus on both internal and external resources chronicled here will also enable scholars and policy makers to evaluate the continued empowerment of stigmatized women with HIV/AIDS.

EXTERNAL RESOURCES

Getting That Monkey off Your Back: Seeking Substance Abuse Treatment and Recovery

It can take a very long while for someone with a substance abuse problem to come to treatment. Previously, some of the respondents felt that they could manage their crack cocaine addiction (among others), and often did so for years while taking care of a family, working, and generally living. It was when they became HIV-positive that their world shifted. They tried many different types of substance abuse treatment programs.

Cynthia, Valerie, Nicole, Billy Jean, Julianna, Daria, Constance, Shelly, Anna, and Simone were women who had previously tried recovery at some point in their lives. They tried to make recovery work this time around. Anna said about the second attempt at recovery, "I knew I was in deep [*raised her hands*] shit. I was scared this time in treatment. I sat up straight at all the meetings, and even tried to be nice to everyone. I really paid attention this time around. I didn't try to get over."

There were many perceived drawbacks in women's minds about treatment. One of the main ones was the sense of confinement. The respondents cited the lack of control over their ability to come and go, the highly regimented schedules, and extensive supervision. With almost all inpatient residential treatment programs, one's mobility is severely curtailed. Inpatient residential treatment programs are an intensive mix of treatment, counseling, group work, and course work within the life skills area. It is a prevailing ideology and practice among treatment centers that being completely immersed in the recovery/treatment process is absolutely essential and effective for substance abusers (see Rapping 1996; Young 1994). Some of the women in my group thought that this was both appropriate and necessary to quitting their addiction.

When the women discussed their initial perceptions about treatment, many of the comments have a similar ring. Another perceived problem with going into inpatient residential treatment was the thought of being "locked up" or confined with many other women. For several of the respondents this was not, initially, an appealing thought. Inpatient residential treatment is often the first institutionalized all-female setting a woman substance user encounters. Most of them come from backgrounds of sex work and drug use, backgrounds that foster competition, and where they have learned to be generally antagonistic toward other women (see Maher 1992).[1] Julianna describes her thoughts about why she first resisted treatment:

JULIANNA: *Mmm-hmm. I wasn't scared, really, of treatment. I was scared of, for one thing I was scared of is my freedom. That is not to be taken lightly. I do not like being confined. And the fact that I couldn't leave this place, and all this stuff, uh-uh. But, I went to treatment. I went to treatment and I hated it. Oh, I hated it with a passion.*

She explains her feelings about entering treatment after discovering her HIV-positive status:

Even though I despised treatment, I decided to try outpatient treatment. It was obvious that I was not doing a good job of taking care of myself. I had the stress of my daughter also to worry about, so I buckled down and went. . . . Parts of it the second time were okay. I learned more.

Robin, after her discovery of being HIV-positive, decided to go to inpatient treatment right away. When I first interviewed her, she said this about treatment:

ROBIN: *This is the first time I've ever been in treatment. The ten years I've been smoking, this is the first time I've ever been in treatment. What made me want to come is because. . . . Well, I had a lot of health problems, by me turning a lot of tricks.*
MICHELE: *Had you heard of HIV before?*
ROBIN: *Yeah. I heard of it, but I really didn't know. But I knew it was bad, you know. And then she asked [a social worker who discussed HIV with her] me did I use drugs? I said, yeah, yes. She said do you want to go to treatment? And I said yeah, so she pulled it off.*

And she took me downtown, and I met Nicole and saw where she works. Her agency made the referral. But I had to make up my mind about treatment on the spot.

But yeah, I said, I want to go. And Nicole asked me if I wanted to be inpatient or outpatient. I said, "No make me inpatient, because if you tell me to come back tomorrow I'm not going to come. I'm not coming." But I told her, I said, "Yeah, it's just best to take me somewhere where I can just stay." I just told the truth. And Nicole took me over here and I've been here since.

I still am kind of in shock, but I'm ready to deal with it. But that's the reason I came to the treatment program. They told me, if I keep on getting high, that with this virus it can kill. I got problems in life, but I don't think I really want to die.

Many of the women discussed that time away from familial obligations, street life, or other problems allowed them to be heard and to express themselves. It was often while in treatment when difficult traumatic incidences in their life, prior to drug use, began to surface and be addressed. For example, Charlene dealt with issues of domestic violence; Valerie, Shelly, Kitt, and Daria (among others) dealt with sexual trauma; Julianna, self-love and acceptance. Frequently, histories of abuse, neglect, and grief come to the surface.

Therapeutic Work on Sexual Abuse

Some of the most striking changes and revelations for some respondents came from the attention and the opportunity to discuss personal and early traumas. These events were overwhelmingly about the sexual violence they experienced at an early age.

Being able to work on these issues constitutes an external resource because counseling was structurally provided by the treatment facility, but it is as well one that leads to the development of internal resources in confronting shame and self-worth issues. This internal resource fully deepens as the women share their experiences with each other and form connections in the HIV-positive community.

It has been noted by researchers that a large proportion of women who are in substance abuse treatment programs have a history of sexual trauma and abuse (see Wadsworth, Sparmento, and Halbrook 1995; Glover 1999). Researchers have also noted that there is connection between the failure to receive therapeutic help for sexual abuse and sexual trauma issues while in a treatment program and later relapse (on withdrawal from programs prematurely Nielsen 1981; on relapse, Barnard 1989; Evans and Schafer 1980; Rohsenow, Corbett, and Devine 1988).

Over half of all respondents had been subjected to childhood sexual abuse. The importance of counseling and, in particular, discussing their concerns with individual counselors was a highly salient theme for respondents.[2] Even if they felt that counselors were not friendly or supportive because of their HIV-positive status, respondents remarked that counselors did a "good job" with helping them discuss past sexual trauma. In prior treatment settings, respondents were either unwilling or unable to discuss such issues. This finding is consistent with the literature on female substance abusers that do not disclose their status of sexual abuse in treatment during the first session (Glover 1999). The possibility of talking to counselors made a difference to many women of whether they stayed within the treatment facility and how they evaluated the treatment they received. In reflecting on their progress, they often remark on the importance of dealing with early sexual trauma.

Therapy is an incredibly salient resource for the women who have been sexually abused and who have had histories of sexual trauma regarding prostitution and drug use. Learning about the frequency and nature of childhood sexual abuse provided respondents an opportunity to make other connections in their lives about structural and material realities.[3] Through this intensive work, many respondents were able to discuss the early stigmatizing effects of sexual trauma. This in turn, I would argue, also lays the foundation for the development of internal resources related to gender and sexuality.

Stigma and Sexual Trauma

Sexual trauma for many of the respondents constituted a stigmatizing characteristic. Sexual abuse made them aware of sexual matters at a young age. In interviews they remarked that early childhood molestation made them feel "different than other girls." They often felt isolated and unable to communicate with anyone about these events. The women who had tried to communicate with another family member and were not believed expressed a sense of invisibility about themselves from girlhood on. It was in treatment, at least initially, that women could begin to understand what role sexual abuse had played in their lives.

Through therapy exploring sexual trauma and on their own, they also began making connections about the consequences of sexual trauma and its possible influence in later life. They became aware of the multiple and complex reasons why women who were abused are specifically vulnerable to later substance abuse. For example, Kitt, said:

> So many little girls who get touched when they're young go on to drink and smoke . . . heavily. That was me. When I found that out, I thought about how vulnerable I was to all the things that have happened to me in life. . . . Thank God I'm alive.

This is important because her finding out information about sexual abuse made her rethink other seemingly "natural" categories:

> When I looked around at who has been molested, I see women who look like me, and went through terrible things like me. All I knew was drugs, that just don't happen

because God wants it to . . . it happens to certain types of people, poor people, people who come from drug users. It happens to little girls by men.

Kitt and others described counseling as providing them with "breathing space" to even begin to understand how early sexual trauma influenced later decisions in life. Being abused made Kitt feel, "worthless, useless, and unfeeling." She said, "It took me to painful places I didn't want to go. But I had to go there. I had to, umm, I had to . . . [*pauses for a long while*] understand what happened to me."

Although, Daria at first did not want to tell anyone about her early abuse, she felt she had to if she was going to be able to deal with HIV. She decided that it was time to "put all the scars on the table." Anna explained it a different way, "It was so freeing to feel like I had several pieces of the puzzle in my hand at one time." Over time, many of the respondents found feminist inspired nonfiction literature on sexual abuse. Daria felt liberated when she found these materials. "It's like a whole new world opened up for me. I felt connected to all the types of women who have been fighting to get our society to see how we allow children, especially girls, to be harmed. I have a much better understanding of how women get lost if molestation happens to them as young girls."

Georgia (who survived an attempted rape) said she used this experience as her "building block." She said that it took her several months to work on these issues and "my reference point kept getting larger and larger. I kept asking questions designed to get at the root of the problem: Why are women abused? Why do we settle for less? Why do some of us begin to prostitute? Why doesn't society address these issues? Why must some of us stay feeling like outsiders?"

Thus, therapy around sexual abuse trauma began to provide a language and vocabulary by which women could start to understand the concept of women as a category, and also helped them to see that other women very much like them (women of color, drug users, lower income) also experienced similar phenomena. It provided them opportunity to see how stigmas intersect and reinforce each other.

Spirituality

One of the features of several treatment programs (especially the residential inpatient ones) that the women credited with helping them through this difficult time was a reintroduction to spirituality and religion. The majority of respondents discussed the central role treatment played in reigniting their interest in spirituality and faith, even if what was being discussed at the treatment center was not to their liking. They found solace in religious and spiritual principles, which gave them hope that they could get through a very troubled period.

Spirituality is not always acknowledged as a particularly important internal or external resource for later participation for HIV/AIDS activists. For the women, however, faith and spirituality were important components enabling them to deal with their addiction and their HIV-positive status. The nature of addiction often poses such challenges that many individuals feel that they must turn over their lives to a "higher power." Some draw on the Twelve Step recovery programs, including Al-Anon (Children of Adult Alcoholics), Alcoholics Anonymous, and Narcotics Anonymous. Cherise credited the spiritual focus in the program as helping her to "jump start" her faith:

> I moved away from the church years ago, because my mom was involved basically in a type of worship that was like a cult. They hated everybody, especially gay people. So I thought I couldn't love God. But being in treatment brought me back to meditation, prayer, and just a deep faith in myself, and that I had the strength to get over this painful period in my life. I draw on all that still.

Valerie found that her particular substance abuse treatment program's focus on religion was too "preachy," but she stated:

> I'm a very spiritual person, but not religious. I don't like people preaching at me, but the religious emphasis did help me to tune into something different than the radio, or television or even the phone. I went and just spent quiet time, and reflected on my life. That was incredibly helpful to me.

The women who are defined as "helpers" tend to draw heavily on spiritual and religious influences. They are also often active in working with local churches in Detroit. Cynthia said this about her experience of spirituality:

> It is the glue that holds me together. Not everyone needs this type of glue, so to speak. I do. My faith is what is helps me get through the day. All the things I'm telling you that I do on behalf of people with HIV, right? All that stuff is possible because I am comfortable being known to God. I don't try to push this on anybody, but anybody who asks why I'm so involved, I have to be truthful and tell him or her what the source is.

Not all respondents are religious or credit spirituality as influential in their decision to be active in their communities. Some see that resource as a limitation; for example, Daria spoke about her feelings:

> The way people use God is very political and sometimes conservative. The God that I was raised with is not who I want comforting me. With some of the programs they got, they really push all that stuff on you. People start looking at you funny if you say you don't believe in God or aren't interested. Most of the women in the community who are doing something positive, they don't try to shove it down your throat.

Facing Stigma in Treatment Centers

Researchers have noted that a wide variety of challenges are associated with HIV-positive people who are also substance abusers, including homelessness, legal problems, financial problems, limited social resources, and mental health issues (Sargent et al. 1999). To date, however, scholars know very little about what types of obstacles HIV/AIDS women face as they access substance abuse treatment. Given previous research on women, AIDS, and stigma, we might suppose that this population faces unique challenges in seeking and accessing treatment.

Even though the women credit recovery as producing several useful and positive outcomes, and I argue that they were able to utilize external resources and develop internal ones, there were many conflicts between HIV-positive women and other women and staff members who were not infected. Stigma from treatment staff and other clients was the major contributing barrier they cited about their care. At the time of the initial research, none of the women had counselors who themselves were HIV-positive even though several respondents had participated in programs with an HIV/AIDS component.

In the last five years, several Detroit substance abuse treatment programs have attempted to incorporate HIV/AIDS information and support for HIV-positive clients. The women's accounts, however, suggest that in many types of treatment centers they faced HIV stigma that often reinforced their initially traumatizing experiences with peers and medical providers. Respondents often felt uncomfortable disclosing their status to counselors, treatment staff, and other women in the program. Respondents contended that some staff members seemed to lack appropriate training or knowledge, or that they displayed bias.

Stigma from Personnel

All but two of the sixteen women cited stigmatizing remarks from personnel in treatment facilities. Incidences of stigma range from casual observations to direct comments about the respondents' HIV status. From the data, it appears that residential treatment facilities posed more challenges; this may be prompted by fears (of both clients and staff) about living in close contact with an infected person.

Respondents mentioned overhearing derogatory comments about them made from one staff member to another. One staff member said, "It's hard to tell with them. She may not get better." Five of the sixteen women cited problems in getting treatment staff to respond to HIV/AIDS related health issues, including scheduling time with doctors or generally putting them at the bottom of the priority list. Women perceived that being HIV-positive was an additional "nuisance" or was "burdensome" to treatment staff. Shelly says she was told it was difficult for staff to "keep up with scheduling for doctors." She says she wanted to respond: "It's not like I was going to Disneyland, shit, I had to see the doctor two or three times a week because of liver problems. I didn't want to have to go that many times." Another respondent observed:

> It was so hard to coordinate [with staff] to see my doctors. There was one point, I had to see three different doctors. The place was real strict about when we could leave and they didn't want to provide transportation [emphatically delivered].

Another respondent was forthrightly told, "Your condition and medical problems make excessive demands on the staff."

Sometimes women were too afraid to request any specific HIV/AIDS counseling; in the majority out of the sixteen cases, it was not available anyway. Additionally, in six cases, a women's HIV-positive status, after being disclosed to a staff member, did not remain confidential in group or therapeutic settings, thus putting her at risk for comments, insults, and in some cases threats from other members in treatment.

All these incidences, the women felt, served to isolate them, distancing them from the staff. To assess how other staff members dealt with insulting incidences (from other clients) of which they were informed, I asked several respondents during follow-up interviews: When people would say rude things to you about your HIV-status and you told staff members, what was the response of the staff members?

Most had reported they did not say anything to anyone about the treatment from staff members. The six who did discuss their treatment with personnel said that their concerns were not satisfactorily addressed. The women often felt that the incident had not been handled adequately even if a staff member had been alerted. "Nothing, they'd never try to intervene or help." Shenna said. "I'd go to my room sometimes and cry and think, God help me get out of this place."

Valerie compared her experience in the first treatment center when she discovered she was HIV-positive, to one of the few centers that counseled HIV-positive women, which she found later. "A world better, I didn't feel like a freak. They [the staff] weren't whispering behind my back."

Stigma from other Members in Treatment

Simultaneously women in treatment also experienced stigmatizing treatment from peers. Some of the behavior ranged from avoidance of the woman whose HIV-positive status was known or insults, aggression, and even overt hostility. Other members in treatment made derogatory comments toward the respondents about the sharing of common use items in the house (e.g., the phone) or even sleeping quarters. One treatment program sponsored a weekly day for kids to come and visit their parents. A respondent told me that another member suggested to the staff member that she (the respondent) be asked to stay upstairs and away from the children during the day of the visit. Respondents also told me that other members in treatment suggested that they not perform certain tasks around the facility (e.g., clean dishes and prepare food). Respondents also reported that other members made complaints about their access to and use of bathroom and showering facilities. One woman says she felt like "target practice" and that she had to endure comments about germs, being unclean, disease from the wrath of God, and other kinds of barbs made in her presence.

Cynthia mirrors other women's comments on the nature of exclusion and stigma regarding the sharing of residential facilities:

Once they knew about me being HIV-positive, I could tell the women were careful if we got food from the same pot. It's hard to describe because you know . . . people weren't like "oh get away from me." But [long pause] *none of the women were too welcoming. It's the little things that when you're HIV-positive you know, you notice. One woman, now that I remember, I know she asked the director of the program if the rest of the women get their meals cooked separately. I don't think that kind of shit would happen now, because for one thing people are more informed . . . but it might.*

It's like I can't breathe or relax, you know? There's someone looking over my shoulder. I don't even know how the women found out about me, but it's like I'm under watch.

The comforts of watching television or playing cards in residential treatment were truncated by the sense that women felt isolated and found it more difficult to participate in social activities that strengthen bonds with their fellow recovery members. Respondents discussed the intangible sensation of feeling apart.

This treatment reinforced feelings of invisibility and marginalization for the majority of respondents. Most, however began over time to use these experiences as a catalyst to consider how they might help other women like themselves if they were in a situation to do so in the future. Nicole says, "I say that it is preparation for the real world. What some women felt in treatment helped some of us become who we are today. If staff act that way and they are college educated then what about other folks?" Some of the women draw on their experiences in treatment to help them stay focused on better meeting the needs of their clients—HIV-positive women. They refuse to ignore the issues of poor treatment. Valerie illustrates this point. "When I became a counselor I talked with them about that there wasn't any HIV programs to train staff. I petitioned them to get people in who could train the staff. That was one of the first things I did when I got active."

Indeed, over time as they became grass-roots activists, their organizing resulted in more thoroughly trained staff in substance abuse clinics in Detroit (Berger 1998).

Learning Advocacy Skills

Another external resource of primary importance is that of advocacy training and education. Most of the women in the deep sample are in some way involved with activities that fall under the broad label of "the advocate" and "advocacy." They were most often exposed to the concept of advocacy at some point during either their substance abuse treatment sessions or attendance at events associated with HIV/AIDS early on.

This term comes from a rubric established through the influences of social work, substance abuse treatment, and HIV/AIDS services (see Hardcastle, Wenocur, and Powers 1997). The concept of advocacy within substance abuse and the general recovery movement has been an idea promulgated to help people with specific and daily life stresses. An advocate helps someone who is struggling to recover from addiction to drugs. Advocacy has enabled a person undergoing stress related to recovery to connect with at least one other person who has gone through similar situations. Women, through the course of various treatment programs, were introduced to self-advocacy concepts. Self-advocacy within substance abuse treatment is rooted in the idea that one must take responsibility for staying drug-free. Advocacy means speaking out on behalf of yourself and others (Hardcastle, Wenocur, and Powers 1997). The role of the advocate in relation to wider politicization is discussed in detail in chapter 7.

Advocacy in the substance abuse context means acquiring a certain set of skills to continue to remain drug-free; if one chooses to, a person can help others stay drug-free. While becoming more involved, respondents later utilized the attention given to concepts such as self-efficacy, interaction with others, and speaking skills. The types of activities that fall under the rubric of advocacy are those that augmented many of the women's existing civic skills (communication, reading, networking).

Advocates may also be social workers or other human service workers who (ideally) help people self-advocate. In the recovery context, they can assist people by encouraging them to attend AA or other Twelve Step meetings, accompanying them to the sessions, helping find employment and secure housing, and easing the general difficulties of recovery. An advocate is a person who will do whatever is necessary to help someone through the long and challenging process of recovery.

Within recent HIV/AIDS initiatives the term *advocate* has been used to encompass a volunteer role, paid employment in city or state agencies, or community groups oriented toward human service work. Paid advocacy typically occurs through monies set aside at the state level from the Ryan White Act and other state funds, enabling states to generate programs that support advocacy and other training for people with HIV/AIDS. The intent is to help newly diagnosed HIV/AIDS patients with basic service support. Advocacy can involve a paid position or nonpaid work, encompassing a wide range of possibilities:

> Advocacy can be used at any intervention level, collectively or separately, and by a professional of any title, even though it is commonly thought of as an activity in which one person goes to bat for another. (Hardcastle, Wenocur, and Powers 1997, 351)

Advocacy in a paid position usually involves client work (case management, educational training, budgeting, administrative or secretarial duties, face-to-face work). Advocacy that involves payment allows women access to institutional support, a modest stipend or salary, and status within the community. Advocates are often associated with an agency, treatment center, community center, and the like, and their work brings them into contact with a wide range of people.

When advocacy moves past traditional expectations into that of group endeavors and defining an agenda (and for our purposes advocacy here contains both paid and unpaid work), it suggests an expansion of the original role. The women have used this label to continue to create and expose group concerns. As Wagner suggests, advocacy often has the potential of transforming "private troubles" into "public issues" (1990, 185). This is an unrecognized category of informal participation for marginalized and stigmatized groups of people. Research on the various forms of advocacy and women's participation in activities (paid or not) remains in the shadows, because (1) it often takes place in physical locations (drug treatment centers, or community centers, or on the "street"), understudied by many social scientists; (2) it encompasses a set of diffused positions involving human service work, which until recently have not been viewed as a connecting bridge into participation; (3) much of advocacy involves skills and abilities that are gendered and often undervalued in society.

Women like Billy Jean and Valerie, among others, who found themselves in inpatient or outpatient facilities that had a specialized HIV-positive component, benefited from the attention given to HIV/AIDS advocacy. Nicole, Charlene, and other HIV-positive activists would sometimes make appearances in various facilities and speak to women about HIV/AIDS. This was in effect to begin the process of peer modeling and learning and of making contacts for the HIV-positive women, although it would be much later that women would have the opportunity to contact any of the speakers.

These programs also informed respondents about the possibility of becoming an HIV-positive counselor later on. Additionally, they were made aware of city and state programs that supported skills-building for HIV-positive women. Other educational forums were made available to these women.

Later, I discuss two respondents who were able to begin their community work outside of the formal structures of the advocacy route. However, for the majority of women advocacy is one of the first ways in which they become connected to resources and learn about the HIV-positive community. Many of them keep an advocate role and even blend it with other types of activism. It will be interesting to see how the dimension of advocacy evolves over the long term as we move into the third decade of HIV/AIDS organizing.

## CHAPTER SIX

Life Reconstruction and Gender

Are you sure, sweetheart, that you want to be well?
—Minnie Ransom

MINNIE RANSOM, a fabled local African American healer known to help women in various states of need, is a prime character in *The Salt Eaters*, Toni Cade Bambara's novel of redemption at both the community and individual levels. As I chart respondents' journey in this chapter, I am reminded that they did not have a charismatic, caring midwife or healer, someone who could assist them to give "birth" to themselves—their female selves—as Minnie does in this powerful novel. She reprimands while she helps, reminding each character that healing is always an individual choice and a process. In choosing to understand what it means to be a woman with HIV, the women of this study made a significant choice that allowed them to help others. In this chapter, I explore the dynamic ways they renegotiated aspects of their gender identity, enlarging it, so to speak, to comprehend and cope with the multiple aspects of being an HIV-positive woman.

Although most of the women went through some type of denial and active drug use after their initial diagnosis, they had to face the fact that they were HIV-positive. Early on they surmised that this would mean great changes in their lives. Georgia, after becoming HIV-positive, said that for years she felt she was floating along and looking for a "lifeboat." She added that she realized at some point she would have to fashion a lifeboat for herself, because there was not one coming. Their work on gender identity constitutes internal resources that were identified, developed, and treasured.

There are two main themes that compose the category of reconstructing gender identity. The first theme is *redirecting HIV stigma related to sex work*. The second theme is *sexual self (re)education and empowerment*,—that is, ways in which women sought to empower themselves around: (1) safe sex and (2) renegotiation of sexual boundaries.

ASPECTS OF RESPONDENTS' GENDER IDENTITY BEFORE HIV/AIDS AND LIFE RECONSTRUCTION

Before we can evaluate how aspects of their gender identity changed, we need to know something about their sense of gender consciousness prior to acquisition of the HIV/AIDS virus. There is great variation in which gender seemed to be a salient category to respondents. From interviews and conversations with respondents, I would argue that for the majority of respondents, their sense of gender consciousness was diffuse. More importantly, their awareness of gender solidarity, or tendency to view themselves as commonly linked with other women, I would argue was low to nonexistent prior to the acquisition of the HIV/AIDS virus.

Some women, when discussing their adolescence, mentioned that their families discouraged high achievement and ambition because they were girls. Others continually cited internal tension and conflict between what they wanted to achieve and the various social pressures they faced, often attributing to the fact that they were female. Billy Jean, Cynthia, Daria, Charlene, and Julianna expressed high degrees of ambivalence about having children, as well as feeling pressured to marry men they did not love.

Although some, in particular—Georgia, Cherise, and Constance—spoke about the influence of differential gendered treatment either in their private lives, or as reflected in society, this recognition did not translate into gender solidarity. If anything, for most of the group, before acquiring the HIV/AIDS virus, they saw themselves *at least* two steps removed from the average woman because of their lifestyles. They often viewed their existence outside the boundaries and scope of traditional values and expectations for women. Their lifestyles tended to transcend and transgress community norms about "appropriate" gender behavior.[1] Most of them did not see themselves as good mothers. Many of their children, at some juncture, had been taken away by state authorities or were living with relatives. Some women identified with "the life," including enjoying drug use, partying, sex work, and occasional criminal activity. They realized that these activities separated them from many of their female peers, female siblings, and female relatives.

The one area where they seemed the most accepting of traditional ideas about what women should want was in the realm of desiring a partner who would take care of them both emotionally and materially. Billy Jean and Shenna strongly expressed this desire.

What makes their latter transformation so worthy of comment is that respondents often had expressed a range of myths, stereotypes, and other negative ideas about being a woman. Given their experiences with street-level sex work and crack cocaine use, they were predisposed to have negative feelings about other women. From the context of their own experiences over time, through the emotional work on their own and with other women, the glacier of some of those assumptions thawed and began to melt away.

These insights should not come as a total surprise. Research and theory suggest that women of color and lower-income women tend to identify and privilege the experience of being a person discriminated against on racial or socioeconomic grounds or both, as opposed to solely identifying with gender discrimination (see Collins 1990; hooks 1984; Hurtado 1989). For some women of color, gender consciousness is often muted and not as strongly emphasized or as well articulated as race and ethnicity consciousness, because of discrimination both at the individual and collective levels.

REDIRECTING HIV-STIGMA RELATED TO SEX WORK

At every step in dealing with the HIV/AIDS virus (from initial diagnosis through treatment), respondents were given particular messages about being a woman with HIV. Many of them discovered, when they *could* get medical help, that medical providers in subtle and overt ways communicated that they did not fit the mold of those who were supposed to be HIV-positive (i.e., they were not men).[2] Women also discovered that peers, relatives, and loved ones held them as being solely responsible for their problems. Additionally, they were constantly reminded that their past histories of sex work and drug use were only a justification for the disease. They often received consistent messages that because of their past behavior they deserved this disease. I argue that all of these events converged to make the women examine what *they* really thought about their prior illicit activities, specifically of sex work. This critical examination would later provide them with the strength and ability to help others who struggled with similar stigma.

Popular notions about the HIV/AIDS lay the burden and the blame on women. This accusation, made to them either specifically as sex workers or as "dirty" carriers of HIV, stems from a long history of the idea of the polluted, diseased, or contagious woman (see Bell 1994; Sacks 1996). They were not among the "worthy victims" of the HIV/AIDS virus which included children, hemophiliacs, or monogamous heterosexual women who acquired the virus from a husband who was bisexual.

Through the process of dealing with the disease, many of them repeatedly expressed their stigmatized status for being former sex workers and being HIV-positive. They recognized, as Christensen suggests, that acquisition of HIV "tends to worsen already existing forms of inequality and oppression based on gender, race and ethnicity, class, sexual orientation, and ability/disability level" (Christensen 1992, 5). Even after several years of activism, women were still sometimes worried about what it meant to speak about HIV/AIDS from a stigmatized background. Anna talked in an early interview about her fear of not being taken seriously by people when she wanted to discuss HIV/AIDS prevention: "Who's going to listen to me? I was on the street half of my life. Cops, people in the neighborhood, even kids think the worst of us [women] who have used drugs and prostituted."

Some of the women, even after going through training and other types of self-empowerment, expressed hesitation when talking to people because of fear of the stigma about how they acquired the disease. Here's one observation:

> SHENNA: *People make all sorts of assumptions about what we "did" to get HIV. In the beginning I felt so ashamed. I didn't want to talk about it with nobody. It was bad enough when people knew I was working on the street.*

Although sex work is a stigmatizing activity, and their lives were affected by that stigma, they also simultaneously possessed lenient or accommodating attitudes about sex work in general. Most women when narrating their sex work histories were careful to distinguish between their drug use and the necessity of street-level sex work or even survival sex versus sex work as an occasional revenue-generating activity. Although they were often severely scorned in relation to previous activities, many of these women did not see those activities as immoral, nor did they feel they should carry the burden of blame for them.

Respondents had multiple and varied experiences with sex work.[3] Women's descriptions of their first exchange of money or material items for sexual services are highlighted here.[4] As some quotations below hint, first sexual experiences with exchanging sex for money were not necessarily a break from their conception of "normal" gender relations. What is suggested here is that for many of them there was not a break in their sense of identity for this activity; if anything, sex work extended the boundaries of what were considered somewhat acceptable relations between men and women.[5]

We begin this discussion with Nicole, who from earlier chapters came to "the life" during a time of experimentation with drugs and sexuality:

> NICOLE: *OK. The first time I turned a trick, had a date was when I was driving my cab. This is funny. The first time, this guy kept on wanting me—another cab driver—kept on wanting to get with me, and so he finally wanted to move in.*
> MICHELE: *Your first date with this other cab driver, how old were you?*
> NICOLE: *Yeah, 22. By this time, I had my regular friend, Doug. But he wasn't my date or anything, I really liked him. And then I met this man, and he was married. And so he would be good to me and everything. He would look out for me. So I ended up just having a regular date. He became my regular date once a week. I'd meet him someplace, and he became my regular date. So that kind of kept me from being wild and loose for a while because I wanted to give him respect, and I didn't want my name to be circulated through the cab drivers like that. And once I stopped driving a cab, I ended up working in a gas station. I was messing around with guys that I met through the gas station, and that was just wild. Because I was really heavy into mescaline then, and it seemed like when I had sex off the mescaline, I would just be going for hours and hours.*
> *And it seemed like I was being underpaid.*

Notice that in Nicole's description her language about her friend who became a "regular date" is used in a specific way: he supported her and there was an exchange of sex for other nonmaterial and material items. She also distinguishes this type of exchange from being on the street and being involved with drugs. We discussed this topic at length:

> NICOLE: *I tried that [walking the street], but you know what? That wasn't me. I was more like the at-home type, and I meet people and I end up having dates. Now I tried it right before I turned 21. I did try it right before I turned 21, down in the Cass Corridor. I remember, I had this little part time job making patch blue jeans. So the guy that ran the place was a pimp, and this guy I was messing around with at that time thought he wanted to be a pimp. And I thought I was in love and I said, "Well, let's try that." But I ended up—I had on these platform shoes and [my feet] started bleeding, I bled for the whole day. I'm so glad I never did get a date like that because I might have still been out there. Once I was on crack, I did it while I was on crack, though, but it was kind of different. I ended up being down here on Woodward by Buena Vista. And the dates that I had picked up, they were kind of nice to me, and stuff. But most of the time I just did it out of my house. I used to sell drugs, and guys would come over and they'd be looking for somebody. And then I would end up going on there with them and smoking their stuff and getting the money. And then [much emphasis] during the last of my addiction, I did some terrible things.*

We turn now to Robin who relates her first experience with prostitution:

> ROBIN: *First time? That's a long time ago. There was an old guy who lived in the neighborhood [she goes into detail about this neighbor]. But anyway, he offered me some money. I didn't think nothing of it. And then it gradually became a part of me. . . . I think I was about fifteen. Fifteen or sixteen, yeah. I wouldn't give my number or name to him.*
>
> *I didn't really think about it too much. He just gave me the money and I took it, and that was it. I didn't think nothing of it.*

Other respondents had experiences similar to Robin's in their early twenties, either experimenting with prostitution on their own, casually posing nude for someone, or working as an exotic dancer. Almost all had some form of exchange of sexual services for monetary or other material items before the onset of their drug use.[6] Constance discusses her viewpoint on this issue.

> CONSTANCE: *Here is what you are asking me. Yes, I liked the work that I did when I was a call girl, especially when I was young. I supported myself and traveled all over the country. No one in my family was the wiser. Even when I wasn't working, I had men friends who supported me. I loved being a nurse, but the money . . . and child the*

flexibility in some of the situations I had was just unbeatable. Also, I worked with some girls down in the Bahamas. That's when I really had to look good, because all those men were on vacation. You know.

Dealing with family members and others (non-HIV-positive people) who were rude and critical regarding their drug use and sex work backgrounds was not easy; as noted before, several of the women relapsed throughout the process: Valerie, Julianna, Georgia, and Shelly. After three months, Robin decided to tell her mother she was HIV-positive. Her mother became very upset, and shouted at Robin. Robin said her mother yelled:

I told you about being in the street! All those men you've been with, this virus could have been from anywhere! How many men did you sleep with? You are a disgrace. How could you do this to yourself and your family?

These early incidences would later become fodder for disagreement, but initially the women alternated between shock and feelings of shame. Later, they responded by learning and educating themselves, and speaking out against perceived injustice. In attempting to understand the multiple levels of exclusion and stigma the women faced I wrote an extended fieldnote in mid-1997:

Because of being raised in New York City and familiar with the struggles of gay people with HIV I thought that I was prepared to understand marginalized women's form of exclusion in my sample. When I began to hear the stories [of various women], they touched me in a very personal way. All of the activism that I had witnessed regarding ACT UP and other radical organizations devoted to destigmatizing HIV and AIDS I regarded as cool, interesting, and important, but remote. Even though I knew a close friend who was HIV-positive, he was living in San Francisco. And he was white, upwardly mobile, possessed an excellent health care plan, and an ever-increasing web of support groups.

When I began to listen to the challenges of these women, I realized that not only are these women the new face of the virus, but that they have the least resources for trying to change institution and societal influences. These struggles grounded in everyday politics, are the framework these women use.

It was a cold day in February when I first went to a small organization devoted to HIV-positive women, New Day for Us.[7] It's a small inpatient residential program that supports women with HIV/AIDS who are struggling to meet the demands of everyday living. The director informed me of several of the fights taking place in the community where their organization was housed. One of the struggles involved the church, which was located right around the block.

Most of the residents within the community supported the house and realized that just because it supported women with HIV/AIDS that it did not mean that drugs, lawlessness, or disease would follow. The preacher in the church, however, had openly said that the women from a New Day for Us were not welcome at service or in the church. He said in many sermons that they were the carriers of disease, had sinful bodies, and should be shunned by the community's congregation. My mouth dropped open when the director relayed this story. I said, "Surely, he can't be serious."

She gave me a stern look. "There are people who want to have nothing to do with these women," she told me. She told me another story about a woman that had been a part of the house for the year. She had developed AIDS and was dying. Her request was to have last rites administered to her. They had to get a minister from another neighborhood, because no one [from any of the denominations] was forthcoming. Additionally, the woman made it known that she wanted to reconcile with her family. Her family refused to travel to Detroit, even when the project director said that the home would pay for the costs. The family even told her they would not claim the body. Thus, when the woman died only her friends from that home surrounded her. (Fieldnote 1997)

Women tried to redirect HIV stigma in relation to sex work in various ways, individually and collectively. On an individual level, they refer to their time on the street as "I did what I had to do." At first one might be tempted to see this as a "grin and bear it" approach. It often helped them to diffuse many of the emotional issues that are connected to the general idea that crack users and sex workers "spread" HIV/AIDS. This sense of acceptance, however, was important in that it allowed them to ask others what they would do in their place. Most of the respondents over time adopted this attitude. Shenna said, "You just have to ask them . . . How would you survive? How would you deal with men who are ruthless? How? I try to break down the ways in which women are vulnerable on the street. Most women won't sell drugs or rob people like the men do. People have their limitations to [understanding] what women can do. We were very creative out there, but when it comes down to it, women on the street face different realities. This is usually not what people want to hear." Valerie's comments echo similar themes: "Would people have preferred that I busted someone's head in so that I could score? That's what the men do, they perform all kinds of terrible acts to score drugs. They also hurt people. I knew women who stole cars, did credit card scams and the like so they would not have to work on the street."

Respondents engaged people in lengthy discussions questioning the distinction between "normal" gender arrangements and prostitution. Several of them had been influenced by the writings of organized, active sex workers in both the HIV/AIDS movement and other movements globally to decriminalize and destigmatize sex work (see Chapkis 1997).

Others, as they became interested in counseling, tried to break the enormous silences around the issue by introducing the topic in support groups for women with HIV/AIDS. Julianna discussed the difficulties she encountered when she wanted to raise the issue of sex work and prostitution in a group she was cofacilitating in a hospital.

> *They wouldn't have it. All I wanted to do was to try to lead a discussion about what every women who was on crack did at some time or another . . . have sex for money. How they felt about it. I can say it, other women I know can say it. See, I started bringing it up because I had to go through so much shit around it, and at the time there were other women I knew who were struggling with the same things . . . in our lives. But because I was a cocounselor, and did not have a degree they basically advised me not to. It was like they were scared that I was going to open a big Pandora's box. . . . That's when I knew there were many things women really couldn't talk about . . . and they . . . we weren't going to get well unless they did.*

Now that Julianna is well established in the HIV-positive community, she is able to incorporate issues of prostitution and sex work into her groups and community-wide discussions.

Georgia related that at several of the workshops for high school students she is asked to facilitate, invariably the discussion about HIV/AIDS leads to the topic of prostitution. She constantly has to dispel the concept that it is women on the street who are "dirty" and who pass it along, or give it to a man:

> *Now kids ain't stupid, and I have to respect that. They might have a cousin, or someone who they've seen on the street prostituting, and stuff like that. They might know someone with HIV. So, I have to be very delicate on all sides with these kinds of issues. I try to talk about how women on the street are not these terrible people. Sometimes, I get so frustrated with them I make us all write a poem on the subject.*

During a rainy and gray afternoon, I watched Nicole during one of her support groups initiate a discussion about the realities of women on the street and paid sex. She wanted to point out behaviors that might have been practiced then, in order to stress they should not be repeated now that some of the women were HIV-positive:

At a group meeting in 1996 the following discussion took place:

> NICOLE: . . . *Okay, our topic is going to get into behaviors, which we still might be doing, from when we used drugs or were on the streets.*
>
> *Now, no one is going to make me feel ashamed for what I did back then, and no one should make you feel ashamed today, ladies. I was doing what half the other women in Detroit was doing. It wasn't all bad, and it wasn't all good.*

Nicole went on to ask the group questions about prostitution:

> NICOLE: *We have all these names for the ladies on the street. What are some of them?*
> [At first the group is silent . . . then two women shout out names]
> FIRST WOMAN: *Ho! Skeezer!*

SECOND WOMAN: *Yeah, Skeezer! Freak! Scuzzy!*

NICOLE: *And we have been them all haven't we ladies?* [Silence . . . then slow nodding by some of the women.]

The group went on exploring, under Nicole's direction, stereotypes about women on the street. Two of the women in that circle talked about having to hear rap music or watch movies that portray extremes of behavior of women on the street. They discussed having to face friends and family with the added expectation that they explain everything to them. At one point Nicole said to the group, "No matter what we did, we still have a right not to be taken advantage of now. We're not on the streets now, life has [now] brought us a new challenge and we must adapt. Tell anyone, anyone who tries to ruffle your feathers about it [that] you are not dirt that you weren't dirt when you were out on the street. Study the contradictions that they give us women in relation to the streets."

Later, when I talked with Nicole about what she perceived as her role in helping HIV-positive women deal with issues of prostitution and stigma:

NICOLE:[8] *I just want to be able to say what I have to say on behalf of the community and behalf of people who are HIV-positive. Especially for women, because a lot of women are still sitting in the house, they're isolated, they're being caregivers, they can't stand up and say they're HIV-positive because they got kids and they don't want their children to be embarrassed or anything like that. They don't want their kids to have to go through that. Either they will look at their mother like she was a crack head or a prostitute, something like that. And they won't look at it like the man gave it to the women and stuff. A lot of women are still in denial about it. They're ashamed, they hurt. All of the above.*

Nicole's comments also mirror other women's concerns that they have to shoulder most of the burden in dealing with HIV. The clients that they engaged in sex for money are not stigmatized; neither are women's partners, who may or may not be HIV-positive. Many of my respondents also felt that Detroit men are allowed to shirk their responsibility regarding the transmission of HIV/AIDS. They were not held accountable for their possible contribution to the current dilemma either through their participation as substance users or as paying participants for sexual services within local drug economies.

Kitt became animated when discussing the assumptions made about women on the street that might have the HIV/AIDS virus. I talked with her after one of her FIT shifts.

KITT: *Lots of people want to blame the "crack hos" for everything. What about the men who use them? The men who are users have just as many problems as those women out in the streets. I know everybody needs help. No one woman is more to blame than another woman.*

Cynthia recounted a disagreement at a holiday dinner. She had been HIV-positive for two years, and her family never wanted to discuss the matter, yet the conversation turned toward criticizing and making assumptions about women on the street:

> CYNTHIA: *Everything is going along fine and good, you know, we're all trying to eat. Turkey's good, macaroni and cheese and everything's good, and then I try to casually bring up something about new stuff I'm learning for HIV. Well, my mother don't even want to hear it. And I'm talking, just in general about the numbers of people in Detroit with HIV. And out of nowhere my cousin Tyrell starts talking about "these dirty bitches" that be spreading AIDS and stuff. And I just put down my fork, and said, "Is that how you think I got it, by being a dirty bitch?"*
>
> *He answers me with something like, "Hey, those girls don't care, on the street they ain't clean." And you know, if I wasn't having HIV and just been like everybody else I wouldn't have paid no mind and probably would have agreed with them. I kept trying to say to him, it doesn't matter how we got it . . . it's about what we are going to do with it. So there went the dinner and the turkey, you know, it really wasn't pleasant no more.*

Talking to Cynthia some time after the family incident we discussed her thoughts on women and HIV:

> *Now, I don't take nothing from nobody. I can get really on the rampage, I don't want to hear about anyone deserving to get HIV/AIDS. My family don't even try to come and play that with me. . . . I'm not meek anymore . . . you know going to let everyone walk all over me because I got this disease. . . . It doesn't matter how I got it. . . . It's here and I'm dealing.*

As some women were able to redirect their own sense of HIV stigma in relation to sex work, it gave them a sense of solidarity and empathy with women who are out there still struggling (both HIV-positive and non-HIV-positive) on Detroit's streets. Robin said, "People can't gang up on you as much when you have better information. Nicole and others really helped me to see that. It's like ladies, ladies, we are all in the same sad and pitiful boat together. But, if we stick together, we just might make it ashore." Daria discussed her way of dealing with assumptions about her HIV status: "See that's why information is so critical. Now, I just cut people off at the pass . . . right before they start into something offensive. I am armed with facts, it's like my web of protection." Kitt, whose community work frequently takes her onto the streets of Detroit, said:

> KITT: *You can be a proud whore. I never was, but women can do it. They can protect themselves from HIV/AIDS, too. I think they shouldn't be on the street, and I tell them that, but a woman can carry herself fine and do a good job. Believe it or not. . . . I just didn't like my job when I was out there.*

The women, it could be argued, through their activities and consciousness raising of these issues become more sex-positive, a term which has been applied to number of progressive (feminist and leftist) strategies in destigmatizing sexual behavior and promoting a wide variety of sexual expression (see Queen 1997). Some of the women who have traveled and read widely utilize these concepts in their work in Detroit in helping others design integrated programs for women with HIV.

SEXUAL SELF-(RE)EDUCATION AND EMPOWERMENT

Although all of the women engaged in sex work and were sexually active earlier than most women, they discovered that becoming HIV-positive entailed approaching sexuality in a very different way. Many of the women, as expressed in interviews, learned little about sexuality from their parents. Women described the embarrassment, shame, or silence they received from parents when they tried to openly discuss sexual topics. As mirrors the wider culture, they found out about sexuality through peers or early sexual encounters. As the women look back at what their lives are like now, they echo Constance's remark: "This is the first time I really know what I'm doing about my sexuality and body." And Kitt elaborates, "Can you believe, after being on the streets all those years? Now I know certain things I'm supposed to feel and how my body works."

The women who discovered their HIV-positive status pre-1992 have demonstrated the most assertiveness in developing this resource of sexual self-education. I believe this results from the fact that they had to seek out information that was just emerging on women and HIV/AIDS. Also, initially in order to do the community work that they did, they had to become well versed in how to reach HIV-positive women about sexual matters regarding their health. Some of this knowledge came from attending out-of-state workshops, creating workshops from the knowledge they gleaned, reading materials, lobbying, and networking with other HIV-positive women.

Overall, the bedrock of sexual self-education rests on the idea that they have had to take more responsibility for their bodies and sexual health, including understanding how the HIV/AIDS virus affects a woman's body differently from a man's body.

Safe Sex

One of the most difficult areas for the women to navigate in their personal life was in the discussion of safe sex. Given their prior experiences on the street this is understandable. Safe sex practices are extremely important in the lives of people with HIV. It is the package of self-knowledge that comes along with being an HIV-positive person.

Sometimes, a woman learned about safe sex to protect her partner more than herself. If the woman was still single then she thought about safe sex for when she would have a partner. Safe sex practices have been documented as difficult for women (both HIV-positive and non-HIV-positive) to negotiate (see Schneider and Stoller 1998). I believe this difficulty is compounded for women who have had problems with substance use. The women learned about safe sex sometimes on their own or through the help of fellow HIV-positive female friends. As some of the women began to feel comfortable in their bodies, they were able to share that knowledge.

> NICOLE: *And when I was first learning [about safe sex], I felt so kidlike . . . I had to be able to say what this was . . . girl, I even teach women about female condoms!*

Julianna discussed her feelings about leading support groups down the same terrain as she had gone:

> JULIANNA: *And the women hate this part, just like I did. They don't want to approach their husband or whatever. It's really hard because they are so used to the men calling the shots in bed . . . and you know out of bed, too. I've seen some good videos which I use to help the women along. But every time I really teach it, I learn things about myself.*

Cherise discussed her experience:

> CHERISE: *Being a lesbian I really wanted to just shrug my shoulders about safe sex, but I knew that wasn't responsible. I had to read a lot because there is some confusing information about what is safe sex for lesbians. But now I'm really into it and into sharing what I know with people.*

Cherise and others designed and implemented safe sex parties/trainings for HIV-positive women, (lesbian and heterosexual) throughout the Detroit Metro area.

The area of relationships is fraught with ambivalence and fear for many respondents as they first began disclosing to intimate partners their HIV-positive status. Women said they had fears and doubts regarding their self-worth as potential mates when first discovering their HIV-status. In repeated interviews a typical answer to What was your greatest fear in being HIV-positive? was, "Being rejected." Women expressed fear around not being able to find a suitable partner, not finding love, being rejected by a man. Many of the women expressed their fear that they might never find a partner. Over time, this assumption underwent degrees of scrutiny.

When a woman becomes HIV-positive, she often undergoes conflict within her primary relationship, if she is in one. If she is still vulnerable to substance use, the moment of HIV/AIDS disclosure and its impact on sexuality becomes a critical moment. Renegotiating sexual boundaries is connected to taking care of one's self sexually. Negative experiences with men in this area have suggested to many of the women that they have to be strong enough to deal with conflict that may arise in relation to sexuality with a potential partner. After disastrous results, to be discussed shortly, often the women realized that they were going to have to be confident enough for themselves, regardless of a partner's response or even having a partner. This process is made even more difficult if the woman was overly male-identified (e.g., being excessively concerned about having a partner, male approval, and the like) or in a physically abusive relationship.

Renegoitating Sexual Boundaries

Several of the women had relapses after they told male partners they were HIV-positive or asked them to use a condom or practice safe sex. These experiences made them more aware of how important it was for them to disclose their HIV status early on, and to have some level of comfort around disclosure.[9]

The rejection of women around sexuality and HIV/AIDS issues is an important one in the lives of struggling HIV-positive women. In order for the women to become effective in their roles as counselor, advocate, friend, and agitator, it took recognition of the intimate decisions women with HIV/AIDS face. Charlene, in this excerpt discussed women's low self-worth in relation to acceptance by male partners:

CHARLENE: *Well, the biggest thing the women I see we now have to deal with is rejection from men. That causes the problems, and leads to a lot of others. I believe if the women would just go ahead on and talk about it, and say forget what the people out there say and live, then we will survive. But we can't survive if we're afraid of what your man is going to say. Afraid of what that man's going to say because I see that every, a lot of women I see, their self-esteem is so low, they put themselves down and feel that they have to be with a man no matter what. No matter if he doesn't want to use a condom! Because [they] think] . . . nobody else would want them. Or, they think it's better to be with a man that's [HIV] infected because he'll understand stuff like that. That's self-esteem, they lose all their self-esteem—they already don't have too much, and they lose the little bit that they have left when they become HIV-positive. That's what I went through, too.*

When a woman is recovering from her addiction and is also HIV-positive, she needs multiple supportive networks of counselors, friends, and families. Women do not often experience these multiple or integrated levels of support. A newly diagnosed HIV-positive woman faces isolation, possible abuse, and the difficulty of telling a partner she is HIV-positive. The times that newly recovering women (with HIV) of the deep sample have relapsed during the life reconstruction process have often been precipitated by rejection and hostility from a partner involving sexuality.

Robin's experiences identify some of the antagonisms that other women face when they disclosed their HIV-status to either a male partner or a trusted male friend. Robin was newly diagnosed, and had not been using drugs for a few months. That day she was upset because she had been shuffled between several different hospitals and doctors in trying to treat a medical condition related to HIV:

ROBIN: *And my second relapse was like three weeks ago. And that was because I had a date with my long-term doctor [physician] friend. I think I've known him about ten years. And he was going to take me out to dinner. But dinner was supposed to be just that in my mind. In his mind it was dinner and motel. I didn't know nothing about the motel part.*

We had fooled around [in the past] but we hadn't always used a rubber. This is a ten-year relationship. So, I felt it was fair to tell him about it [her HIV-positive status]. So I got the nerve up to tell him. And when I told him he just blew up at me. He called me every name in the book: dirty bitch, skeezer, he even said he would never sleep with me again. He made me feel so terrible, so low. . . .

So everything was going bad that day. And then when he came and that happened, I just couldn't take it no more. I felt like my whole world caved in on me. So I went to go talk to my girlfriend, then I just wanted go talk to her. And not thinking that she was selling drugs.

MICHELE: *You just wanted to see her—*

ROBIN: *I wanted to see her and talk to her. Then when I got there and got to talk to her, and all these people coming in, and I said, Oh, man, that's right, she's selling drugs. And that craze hit me and I did it. I stayed out that day. But I only smoked that day, that Saturday. Then I felt guilty all Sunday. I tried to call Nicole all day . . . but I couldn't reach her. But see I'd been clean for about a month and a half.*

Then I just got so frustrated with the tension, the rejection and stuff. And I couldn't even get high because my head was killing me.

MICHELE: *This guy knew you used drugs?*

ROBIN: *No, he didn't know any of this. So I guess it was a shock to him, too. You know, well I told you I had two lives. Yeah, he was all right with that. But when I told him about my virus, it's like he lost his mind. I'm like, OK, be upset but damn, we've got ten years between us.*

Later reflecting on this experience she continued:

Well, I was hurt. It still kind of bothers me. You know, because, I'm looking at the future, it would be kind of hard for me [to be single for a long time]. Because, I was used to having some kind of man in my life. And now that I look at, that's one thing that I don't have, and it's going to be hard now, because by me having this virus, you know. It's the law that you know that you have it, and if you go out and have sex with a guy and they contract it without you telling them, they could take you to jail.

Cynthia, Shenna, and Billy Jean all had troubling experiences regarding dealing with male partners.

> SHENNA: *Well, I had met a man whom I really liked. This was like two years or so ago. Now I knew that I really needed to discuss all that stuff about HIV and sex, but I wasn't strong enough. I couldn't believe he was with me and he knew I was HIV-positive. I was so grateful for that. . . . I wasn't with my husband any longer, and he wanted nothing to do with me because of the HIV. This guy at least tried to act like it didn't bother him. So, on the night we were supposed to have sex, now we had talked about stuff a little, he was acting really funny. He said he didn't want to have a "latex girlfriend." I told him we could try a blowjob with a condom . . . that was safe, but he wanted me to give him one without it, just to prove that I cared about him [long pause]. I'm sorry to say that I did it. He did some stuff to me, not intercourse, but what we did wasn't safe. Then he broke it off the next week, and said he couldn't handle it. He said every time he thought of sex with me he didn't want to think of "germs." Of course, I felt very very dirty. I drank . . . I didn't smoke crack, thank God. I wanted to. . . . I drank some whiskey and stayed high for at least three days. I learned from that experience.*

Although these experiences speak to rejection, the women undergoing them actually come to participate more fully in their own sexual health and sexual identity. They begin to value other aspects of their life regardless of their relationship status. This in turn has motivated some to work on HIV-positive women's issues within relationships.

DEVELOPMENT OF A PUBLIC VOICE: WHAT IT MEANS TO BE A WOMAN WITH HIV

The development of what I am calling a "public voice" is one of the tangible outcomes of the process of life reconstruction. The process of deciding to live with HIV,[10] and then organize with other HIV-positive women meant for my respondents a decision to accept the gendered and political ramifications of being a woman with HIV. For respondents this process was actualized through the activities and roles they embraced. The term "public voice" best encapsulates the process of creating a public identity or persona that interacts with the outside world. This step of naming and claiming an open persona forms the bridge to political activity. This section explores the context of what it means to develop a public voice and the various components that make it possible for women to exercise their public voices. At the end of this chapter, I reflect on a woman who is not able to sustain her political activities because she has been unable to sustain a public voice, which is in part related to her conflicted relationship to gender roles and expectations. The woman's story provides sobering evidence of the transition through these identifiable phases in life recon-struction that was not sustained.

Scholars within the social movement literature have discussed the im-portance of collective identity versus individual identity as a basis for orga-nizing (see Naples 1998; Sudbury 2001). The idea of "public voice" was a salient and repeated data point in my observations and discussions with the women. My investigative mapping of public voice suggest that it exists as a manifestation along a continuum in which collective identity can be expressed. Additionally, although the idea of collective identity is not new, my focus on how this population situates itself in the public realm through a public voice is different from what other scholars working on HIV/AIDS and social movements have identified. There are three areas that I draw on to tease out this broader idea of voice. The first is the feminist articulation on the notion of self and the importance of voice (both as a metaphor for women's experiences and its translation into the material world) (see Olsen 1979; Rich 1979). To develop a strong "voice" has been a concept in theo-ries about women's emotional and psychological development (see Belenky et al. 1997; Gilligan 1982) Second, there has been an emphasis within multi-racial feminist movements to use one's voice both literally and symbolically in the struggle against inequality (see Anzaldua 1990; Speed-Castillo 1995; Collins 1990; hooks 1989; Moraga and Anzaldua 1981). And lastly, the HIV/AIDS empowerment literature has stressed visibility and voice (see The ACT UP/NY Women & AIDS Book Group 1992; Lather and Smithies 1997; Schneider and Stoller 1995). Respondents publicly claim an identifier and suggest to other women they can partake in this collective identity. This does not mean that every political moment is lived under "a woman with HIV" banner. However, it provides them a platform to speak from; embracing a public voice allows them to organize for change. Also, as the term "voice" suggests, respondents acknowledge that they have to speak about their own experience with HIV/AIDS.

What signaled to me the development of this public voice were the ways in which women repeatedly used the phrase "what it means to be a woman with HIV."[11] For some respondents, this reference was no more than a casual phrase used in a longer personal account. Over time though, I observed that the majority of respondents used the phrase often and with emotional clarity, urgency, and vigor. It became part of a larger set of statements and meanings about the self that they used in formulating their tasks within their communities.

Developing a public voice is a culmination of the redirection of the stigma discussed earlier. Those with a public voice can answer questions, speak for themselves, and are no longer so afraid and tyrannized by their pasts. Public voice does not denote merely the ability to speak to a group of people, but to *want* to be engaged about being an HIV-positive person. Respondents see themselves as representatives, and assume the responsibility such a role requires. The following quotations are examples of respondents' sense of responsibility:

NICOLE: *Mmm-hmm. And also it's like, the way I see it is that the women are in so much denial. And then, too, it's not so much about denial, it's that they couldn't stand up and say that they was HIV-positive. Like now, I tell them, I say, "I'll sure be glad when somebody else comes on board that can stand up publicly, you know, all over the United States and say that they're positive from the state of Michigan." Because the ones that we do have speaking, they're limited to where they can speak at, so that their children don't find out, their family members don't find out. I have clients now that say, "Well, I don't want anybody to know." And I'd be like, "OK, nobody will know, but in case of emergency, if you got real sick, I would still not tell nobody your diagnosis, but who can we call in case you get sick?" My thing is that I like to see change and I like to see it for the better, OK. Right now as far as agencies are concerned and stuff like that, and in the government, the government is always changing their mind. One day they say that people with HIV are not disabled, and the next thing they want to do is throw all people with HIV out of the military. You know what I'm saying? And so they're always changing their mind. I like to be part of the movement for change where they look at people with HIV as being human. Just like regular people, quit stigmatizing us, and that's one of those things on there. I've always said that ever since I've started going out speaking. I said, HIV is not what's really killing us, it's what, the way the media portray people being HIV. I told them, I said that I was so glad when I went on my first TV interview, because I stood up and I said, "You see how big I am? They're going to go and find the worst looking person that didn't lose all that weight from HIV from crack probably, and say that person—they want to show that person as having HIV. But they need to keep showing [healthy] people, reinforcing that people are living, people are living, and people are living longer.*

JULIANNA: *See, we [her agency] don't let people continue to be ignorant. I mean, it's kind of a personal thing. If I hear the slightest bit of misinformation about something I try to correct it. And you know, it's empowering to know what you're talking about. Just find out. You can't hide it, you can't put your head in the sand over it. It's almost politically incorrect not to be empowered these days. You just can't sit around and let this happen to you. It's OK for people who are newly diagnosed, have their little mourning period. But you know, you got to get on the bandwagon. They really do. So, they are definitely, more empowered. They're taking more control. And people, especially women are being trained a lot, you know, trained to you know, just get out there and bring other people. From all kinds of organizations and just from each other as well.*

Valerie said the following at a local fundraiser for with PWAs (people with AIDS):

There is something wrong with this country that HIV-positive people are treated poorly. There is not something wrong with you. It's something wrong with our government today. Don't believe the media, please don't believe just the media. HIV-positive people are everywhere from all walks of life. Our lives must be respected.

SHENNA: *When I talk to men who are HIV-positive it is like talking to a different species sometimes. Our issues are different. They might have shame about the disease, but it is coming from a different place. There are more responsibilities on the women. The self-love an HIV-positive woman needs to have to become active on these issues seems different to me than for men.*

CHERISE: *For me to stay politically active, I have to remember what it means to be a woman with HIV.*
MICHELE: *What does that mean, to be a woman with HIV?*
CHERISE: *It means for me to remember that for everything I do, there are women who are going to die because they did not get the right services, the right treatment or who don't know they are infected. I have to stay connected with women's lives, with my own life. I have to stay connected with the reality of the disease for women that I meet who are sick and can't get to support groups, rallies, or meetings. They are still invisible.*

HIV as Empowering Experience/Learning to Like Other Women

Every aspect of their lives respondents connected with being a woman who was HIV-positive. Their tenuous but primary identities were constellations that revolved around the categories of mother, worker, daughter, sister, partner/companion, girlfriend, wife. All of these defining spheres were shattered and reshaped through the gender component of life reconstruction. For some women, it gave them the opportunity to clean house with important people, confront past sexual trauma, violence, and old emotional and physical abuse.

After much emotional work over time, the women move toward wanting to connect with other women and men about HIV/AIDS. HIV/AIDS is identified as a condition that has given them something back, despite all that it has taken.

NICOLE: *All over the United States. During my first three years of me being delivered from alcohol and drugs, I went all over the United States. It seemed like every time there was a conference about HIV and AIDS these two ladies that I call my guardian angels, they, I would ask them, I said, "Would you give me a recommendation letter so I can be able to get a scholarship to go?" And they said yeah, and they did and I ended up going. And one of the things that I wrote down on there that I helped facilitate a women's support group. These women are in denial and I said, unfortunately they don't want to come to the conferences, but I want to attend. And I said, the information that I get from the conference, I will bring it back and share with them. And that's what I did.*

JULIANNA: *We were networking to see ways the different communities were doing things for us to bring back. And you know, figure out how to fill in whatever gaps there are in your program. Fortunately for us, I only see one gap for mine. I did, I did find one gap. But a lot of people have a lot of major communication problems. So, we're pretty much on the path. We're doing real good. Yeah. And I was never able to see it from the national perspective until I met some other women around the country. So we are, we're doing real good. Everything's in place now, we just have to work at it.*

Respondents' ability to like and trust other women is crucial in this discussion. Respondents saw women, prior to their acquisition of the HIV/AIDS virus as not trustworthy, supportive, or kind. The phrase "I couldn't stand to be around other women before HIV" was a common response women gave when asked about what they felt about women.[12] The transition women make is one from distrust and disliking other women to one of appreciation, respect, and camaraderie. Slowly, through networks, support groups, and community work, women peel away those antagonistic layers and develop strong bonds. There is a valuing of the female self that translates out to valuing and validating other women.

Charlene said this about women:

After being in treatment and going what I have gone through with HIV, you try to help a sister out as opposed to always putting her down. I really learned that. You know? It's like workable sisterhood.

Shelly offered her reflections on female friendship:

I have more friends than I used to. Because I used to be popular, but that was the dope. It was me, I hated my own self and blamed it on somebody else. But when I went home to my male friend, I told him, I said, "Women don't like me, they never want to get along with me." It was always me, I had to go through a lot of things to get along with women. Now I can live around my own sex. I used to think I had to have a man friend, because women don't like me. You know, and that was my attitude. Now I can be around women, and I enjoy having women that I can talk to on the telephone, you know as a friend, as well other types of things which involve the work and speaking I do. They call me. It feels good to have a female friend, because in my addiction, no other females wanted to be around me.

There are many different factors that have aided respondents to trust and respect other women, thus paving the way for further interactions and connections. I asked all respondents questions about their perception of feminism. Many of the women did not know what the word meant, and others said for sure they were not feminists. This is not surprising: most American women do not identify with the label of feminist yet when asked about questions of equality their answers (from respondents and many women) typically are in concurrence with other broadly constructed feminist ideas and agendas. Despite this, however, they *do* have working ideas about the utility of women helping each other as best exemplified by

Julianna's long quote. Notice how she moves from a common perception of feminism, one rooted in popular culture, to a more meaningful discussion about everyday relationships with women.

> JULIANNA: *When I think of feminism, the first thing that pops into my mind is Jane Fonda* [much laughter from interviewer and respondent]. *As* Barbarella *[the movie made in the 1960s]. Every time I think of feminism and Jane Fonda, I mean, I remember that* Barbarella. *You didn't think you were going to be a feminist, did you honey, when you did that? But, anyway I think feminism, for real, feminism to me, even that definition in my head has changed. From you know, burning bras to sisterhood. Sisterhood. Let's stop being mean to each other. You know, we do more harm to ourselves than men can ever do to us. Because see, we can rule them if we so choose. We're just not as vicious as they think we are. You know. And I just think that feminism, that the basis of some real feminism should just be sisterhood. Let's take care of each other. Let's stop, you know, [saying] her hair looks better than mine. Well, why don't you go over and help her do her hair better, instead of talking about her? Why don't you lend her that fly outfit that you know she can't afford to buy? Why don't we help each other to feel better? And if we feel better, if we help each other take care of our kids and stuff, you know, life will be a lot smoother for us. They're [men] not going to do it. Men are not going to do it. You know, if we get any help, it's going to have to be between each other. And I just really wish we could do that. It's funny you should ask that, because for some reason, a major issue in my addiction was I was accused of not liking women. And that I didn't like myself, and that's why I didn't like women or some such something. And it may have been true, you know. And I thought about it, and the fact just flashed when you said feminism, that I find that odd that because now, I'm very much, you know, just help the sister out. Because we're all, we're all in the same line. And that includes white women, you know. They may have some things easier, but they're getting squished from the male to female kind of thing just like we are. OK.*

Respondents have traveled to other places and met other women; sometimes these are brief encounters and other times they are more substantive. Among the women who traveled, getting to know women across states (and even countries) was a great source of pride, encouragement, and excitement:

> NICOLE: *Oh, girl, yeah. Oh. I'm talking especially in Georgia and New York. There's some bad sisters out there advocating. And one of the things, and I'm telling you, I like them girls and I like their style because they don't mind speaking their mind, they got their stuff together. And I was like, I'm going to be down just like that. And I am down just like that. And especially in Georgia, they are so together. Michigan has come a long way as far as women and children and they're really trying to recognize women and children more now. But I remember last year, I was just dogging Michigan out. Especially ——— Committee. I was like, in Georgia, they're not scared to say nothing, especially to the government. They will go up on the government's doorstep and tell them how they feel. And they don't worry about no money. And I say, the*

government loves them. And don't the government keep giving them some money? When I brought an issue to ——— the first thing everybody was talking about on the committee, they'd say, "Well, we got to worry about our jobs and stuff." I say, Damn a job. We're talking about people's lives. We're talking about women with children who need this help.

Robin: *I had to examine the ways that I thought about other women, I really did. No one ever taught me to stick up for myself let alone other women. Sisterhood is critical when it comes to HIV. I try to stress that for women who are out in the streets, even though they may not have that mentality now. It's a positive thing to work with other women for me right now.*

Consequences of Not Developing a Public Voice

The importance of this process is made more salient by a brief comparison to Billy Jean's ongoing challenges. Her difficulties with issues of addiction and valuing herself provide insight about other women (specifically Anna) who also struggle with their partner's and others' gendered expectations of them. Her story sheds light on the gendered ways in which HIV-positive women who become and want to remain active are thwarted. Recall, from chapter 2 that Billy Jean struggled with her family's and her own expectations of being like a "normal woman," which meant married with children, and middle-class status. She had many problems trying to fulfill that dream for her family and for herself. Although there are aspects of that ideal which appealed to Billy Jean, she had also voiced a high degree of ambivalence about pursuing certain goals connected to that ideal.

After becoming HIV-positive, she seemed as if she was on the road to life reconstruction. She went through drug treatment, though for a much shorter period of time than other women. She also threw herself into a variety of advocacy activities and spent a brief amount of time at a special program for recovering women with HIV/AIDS. Early on in her work she characterized herself as someone who was committed to change for herself and other HIV-positive people:

I'm an outspoken person, and I live with HIV/AIDS. I'm not ashamed of it, and if I can help one somebody out there to see that this disease don't have to take you away . . . you just don't have to lay down and take it, and that you can prevent yourself from subjecting yourself to running away with drugs, then I'll be happy, you know.

Billy Jean took a volunteer position at Hope for Us,[13] an organization that works with HIV-positive people. She enjoyed these activities and often also helped Nicole with advocacy activities related to women and HIV/AIDS issues. In one interview, she reflected on her progress about life choices. She had decided to get her current marriage annulled. In this passage she clearly articulates her goals about wanting to be of service, and also thinking through the life she does not want:

> *Probably what I'll do is get involved in some more kind of community work through the AIDS community, and keep busy. See, that's what happened when I came home the first time. I stayed home and played homemaker. You know, my mind was always idle, you know, the idle mind is the devil's workshop. So now I plan on staying busy, and with keeping my son, going to these [activities], I pretty much got a structural day planned ahead of me. I plan on giving back something, from what I learned, and that way I can keep focused, yet still be on the issues of HIV in helping somebody else in different areas. So I pretty much know what I want to do, and it ain't based around going home trying to please somebody else. It's about pleasing me today, and making me whole. Because see, I got to live for me. And in order for me to live for me, I have to live for my son. I got to love me today, and I love me today. And get in touch with my spirituality, because ain't nothing out there for me. Ain't nothing out there in those streets for me no more, you know, but a bunch of pain, heartache and headache. . . . I want to be responsible. I've learned so much from everyone else, now it's my turn to give back. I'm really good with people* [emphasis added].

The next interview I conducted with Billy Jean took place about two years later. Billy Jean had relapsed several times since we had spoken. She also got married to a man partly because he accepted her as HIV-positive and seemed to be a good provider for her and her son. Throughout the next set of interviews, when talking about her relapses she tried to construct a frame about her laziness and not being an obedient wife.

However, with an attention to the tensions in her life around gender conflicts, it is possible to interpret her remarks in a different context. Instead, they could also be read as a tension between her partner being threatened of her newfound independence with HIV/AIDS work and Billy Jean's constraints in her new role of wife. Her husband asked her to stop working and stop volunteering, specifically on HIV/AIDS related work. Moreover, ignoring her desire to remain financially independent, he asked her to sell everything and start anew with him.

It became evident in interviewing Billy Jean that she had moved away from her earlier commitments to HIV/AIDS work, not only in spirit, but also in the ties she had maintained with other active HIV-positive women. She also had fallen back on the fail-safe narrative as "women as untrustworthy" to explain her changes. She discussed her new female friends. The women she met in her new role as "wife" and "churchgoer" reaffirmed more traditional gender roles, roles that she already had expressed some conflict with:

> *Well, you know what, most women that you deal with, they have an ulterior motive. If it ain't no personal gain to them, they don't want to be bothered with you. So yes, I would say*

I'm still somewhat a loner. Only I cling to people with a little more spirituality. Women that are stable in their homes. I hang out with the women in church, the old timers. That's what I do. I don't cling to this [waves her hands around room] *because it don't last long. . . . You try to hang on, but some obstacle always comes in the way. If it ain't a man, it's another girlfriend. If it ain't another girlfriend, it's the children. And in reality there's no guarantee that it will go other than us seeing each other coming back. And most of us, out of a handful, will come back. See, I committed to coming back for a year now. So if you're ever going to find me, this is where I, I won't be here, but I'll be down at the* ———— *. And I had started, I had worked for nine months. But it just, it just, I stopped going. Because my husband was like, everywhere we go, you're talking to somebody about HIV. And this is what I want to do.* I wanted to do advocacy work. [Mocking her husband] *"Well, everybody you see, they got to be a recovering addict or someone with HIV," and da da da da. I said, Well, in order to keep what I got I have to give it away. Well, I stopped giving it away. So you know what happened? I lost it* [emphasis added].

What I think she meant when she referred to her comment "giving it away" is her information and help on HIV/AIDS issues. Although she attributes her relapse solely to drugs and social pressure, it could also be surmised that she has a partner who undermines her. Partners of some of the women have questioned their motives around HIV/AIDS work, whether it was taking overnight trips designed to put HIV-positive women in touch with each other, attending rallies, or visiting incarcerated people. Sometimes partners will bring up a woman's past sex work history and suggest that they do not feel comfortable with them going back to places where they were sex workers. Respondents' partners often worry about a woman coming into contact with other men and recovering users. Not all of the partners are easily labeled abusive; rather, their attitudes suggest the gendered nature and understanding of "appropriate" public spaces for women to conduct certain types of activities. This is symptomatic of recurring issues regarding women in the public sphere of politics versus the private sphere of the home (Flammang 1997). Billy Jean's husband enthusiastically encouraged church activities or occasional attendance at support groups. This suspicion interferes in the creation of a public voice. Billy Jean reflects on her husband's behavior:

Plus, he just got all up in arms, said talking about HIV/AIDS made him uncomfortable, and I need to get a new hobby. Plus, the traveling, he didn't like the traveling . . . so it was just all of those things together, so I'm just biding my time, waiting until things die down a little bit. I know what I like to do with my life, and HIV-work is a part of that. Sharing is a part of that.

If we are not careful, her narrative could be read as a woman who "loved too much" or as a narrative solely about drug abuse ("the crack made her do it"). Instead, her narrative can serve as a specific lesson about the multiple barriers faced when stigmatized women try to act on their sense of empowerment. Despite these problems, Billy Jean in one of our last interviews repeatedly reaffirmed her commitment to advocacy work:

> *I'm just starting over again. I'd like to see some of my long-term projects that I was working on women with HIV who have kids started. I went to the memorial display, the AIDS Quilt project in Washington last year. And I'm still on the* ———— *committee. My husband will understand soon that I'm in this stuff for the good.*

Life reconstruction describes a process enabling respondents to become aware of and utilize external resources and develop internal resources. The resources that were gained provided both tangible and intangible benefits. Recovery was a necessary component to later self and group empowerment. Through recovery the women were often introduced to therapy that allowed some to deal with issues of sexual trauma. Additionally, embracing spirituality helped some women through the difficult periods of recovering from crack cocaine use. In recovery, sometimes they were introduced to other peers as role models. Additionally, they were connected with support groups and also discovered city and local funding which helped HIV-positive women.

Although the collectivity of the life reconstruction process can be thought of as a set of nontraditional resources, they do have some commonality and overlap with features of traditional resources like time, money, and civic skills. The recovery process allowed many respondents a certain amount of time (if even only for a few hours for those who primarily went for outpatient treatment) that allowed reflection. Additionally, although the life reconstruction process did not allow for respondents to pursue higher education, many were able to better develop their civic skills through advocacy programs. Finally, respondents' ability to move between paid and unpaid labor helped provide nominal amounts of money.

These processes allowed them to shape different avenues of awareness in relation to their own subjectivity. They were over time able to reject both the narrative of "HIV/AIDS female victim who will die" and "unworthy crack user/prostitute." They were able to forge new aspects of identity using their public voices. They found their ability to speak at first on their own behalf, and then later speak with authority about "what it means to be a women with HIV."

## CHAPTER SEVEN

Making Workable Sisterhood Possible:
The Multiple Expressions of Political Participation

*There is something wrong with this country that HIV-positive people are treated
poorly. There is not something wrong with you. It's something wrong with our
government today. Don't believe the media, please don't believe just the media.
HIV-positive people are everywhere from all walks of life. Our lives must be
respected. I'm committed to finding political ways to get that respect.*
　　　　　　　　　　　　　　　　　　　　　　　　—Valerie, thirty-five

THUS FAR in the discussion, the ways women have used their intersectional
experiences of HIV/AIDS to transform their personal lives has been central. This chapter centers on the political participation for respondents.
The first section of this chapter delves into the range and meanings of the
activities that lead to empowerment on behalf of themselves and others,
thus bringing the study full circle. It introduces the concept of roles as a
useful way in conceptualizing the scope of participation. It also explicates
how the roles of *activist*, *advocate* and *helper* are constituted as blended and
overlapping roles, allowing women great fluidity in pursuing their goals.

Their participation offers a rare opportunity to examine the experiences
of stigmatized women involved in both formal and informal political activities. Due to their often multiple locations as human-service workers, sometimes paid by agencies, and as unpaid caretakers in their communities, the
women are in unique positions to redirect and redefine local struggles,
and create an HIV-positive community. Their self-defined community is
primarily the HIV-positive community: women, men, children, families,
drug users, and prostitutes. They utilize their knowledge and paid positions
as resources for ongoing community struggles.

The second section highlights the features that characterize their participation. It is argued that blended role participation helps to create learning
opportunities that are often experiential, black-female centered, and community oriented as central features of respondents' participation.

THE WOMEN'S DISTRUST OF CONVENTIONAL POLITICS

In beginning the discussion about the meanings of the women's activities,
it is important to explicate the distrust and repugnance of the political

realm that most women espouse. In doing so, I hope to represent some dominant images of politics that may also coincide with how other Americans feel about politics. First, most of the women do not identify the work they do in "traditional political terms." The majority of the women do not call themselves activists or "political people," or view themselves as trying to advance complex "agendas."[1]

Their distrust of the political realm exists in primarily three areas: distrust of public institutions, distrust of coalition building, and distrust of becoming "a political person." The first two areas of distrust are centered in ideas about the ability of people within institutions and groups to honor and recognize them (as HIV-positive women) without distorting or diluting their efforts. The last area of distrust of the political stems from their distaste about what it means to be "a political person." Being a political person, to many respondents, means being someone who is in a weakened position, someone who has to rely on other people to help her. Usually those other people are often people who are seen as having more influence, status, and cachet in wider communities. A political person is also defined as someone who is potentially "out of touch" with the HIV/AIDS community or who cares more about personal advancement than group conditions. There is ongoing internal and community conflict among respondents about personal versus professional/political advancement and serving the interests of the larger HIV-positive community.

For respondents, as primarily women of color with HIV, the political world is often constructed as being dominated by European Americans (specifically men) with perceived institutional power and resources. Professionals who claim to have expertise and authority over them because of their education or professional activity also dominate it.

This distrust permeates their feelings toward public institutions. Advocates in particular are suspicious and continue to be suspicious of the larger public institutions, which they have to now interact with on behalf of themselves or clients including: the medical establishment, city agencies, the criminal justice system and state sponsored task forces. It is understandable, given the experience of respondents, that the women tend to be critical of the political realm. As people who have experienced intersectional stigma, many of their experiences with institutions have been negative. Also, the majority of women did not associate politics as central to their lives before becoming HIV positive. Additionally, most respondents did not come from backgrounds where their parents were active in varied types of political and public institutions.[2]

Before the onset of the virus, the majority of women were not active in their communities, except perhaps in church activities. From the interview material, it is quite possible to conclude that women received negative messages from parents about the political system.[3] They are members of groups in society who often do not have opportunities to politically participate, have lacked adequate resources, and have less reason to believe institutions will help them achieve their political goals and ideals.[4]

"Government" is a catchall phrase, used by some respondents to refer to public institutions. It is a broad and often not well defined term among respondents. Constance illustrates this point when she recounted her experience participating in a study at a nearby university. The study was a longitudinal one of women with HIV/AIDS; the study had government funding. I asked her what her thoughts were about participating in that study:

> *No, I don't think* they're *dumb, but I feel like, I think that* they *know all these things are going to happen, by* them *studying us for all these years. . . . So* they *want to know things from so many women,* they *only allow so many women in the study,* they *know these things are going to happen to you, but* they *want to see how you deal, you know, and everything. It's some of those things, but it makes me angry because* they *know what is happening, and I feel that* they *have these medications, and* they *have these things, and* they're *not giving it to the public.* They're *not giving. Every year* they *come out with a little something else to kind of keep you lingering on.* [Emphasis added]

Then I ask "Well, do you think in your lifetime, they're going to see a cure [for HIV/AIDS]?"

> *No, maybe when my three-year-old grandson's twenty-five or something, maybe we will, and I'll be long gone then. You know. So I get very upset about this.*

She uses the words *they* and *them* frequently throughout the passage, which could stand in for a variety of actors: researchers, the government study, or scientists who work for vaccines and cures to combat the HIV/AIDS virus. Often the words *they* and *them* stood, for many of the women, for representatives of public institutions that compose the "government" including the Detroit Department of Health, city and state agencies, and the court system.

This negative notion about government/public institutions is pervasive. One of the women in the sample of sixteen has espoused ideas that would fall into the category of "conspiracy theory." For example, she believes the government already has a cure for the HIV/AIDS virus and is holding out for as long as it can to get rid of "undesirable" types of people.[5] Some elements of this distrust remain at the surface level, and other elements are more complex and deeply rooted. This deeper distrust makes the women incredibly guarded when they do have interactions with representatives of various governmental agencies. For example, Daria has in the past said, "I always record everything that I do and say after a meeting. You have to. *They* will bury you in so much damn paper and waste time to retrace your steps. *They* have all the time, and money on their side. And you can't forget about the money." There is a pervasive sense that respondents must remain vigilant in their undertakings with "government" people. Their experiences as women with HIV have often put them into contact with representatives of institutions who have at times tried to delegitimate their right to know about their bodies and the validity of experiences of people with HIV. Other political actors, often with more authority, constantly challenge respondents' ability to know and speak on behalf of themselves and other people.[6]

The second area in which distrust of the political process emerges is through respondents' attitudes about coalition building. Coalition building, in the political sense, is an act of trust—recognition that two or more parties with sometimes differing interests can have common goals and agendas. Coalition building helps to combine the resources and strengths of participating members. One of the ways in which political work typically gets accomplished (particularly for) "outsider groups" is through coalition building.

On the one hand, many women realize that coalition building is a useful strategy in reaching stated goals and establishing new ones. There are several potential coalition members in the struggle around HIV/AIDS issues in Detroit; some are city agencies, community organizations, state- and city-appointed task forces; others include mobilized HIV-positive communities (e.g., white gay men). On the other hand, coalition building can dilute the goals of some members. Some of their suspicion and reservation, about alliances, however, is rooted in the idea that people with HIV need to carve out specific and autonomous spaces.[7] Aligning themselves with other groups is advantageous, yet many women feel coalition building "waters down" their priority interest. Moreover, when some of the women, professionally or otherwise, do lend a hand (or advocate coalition building through their paid work), they often feel other groups do not respond in similar fashion to *their* needs.

The women often find coalition building to be an arena fraught with conflict. In trying to get their populations recognized, they encounter inordinate amounts of discriminatory beliefs. Coalition building with white gay male organizations has, in particular, frustrated some respondents. Fieldwork notes suggest that coalition-building efforts often highlight the boundaries between stigmatized and nonstigmatized people working on HIV/AIDS issues. Fieldnotes also document several-coalition-type meetings that respondents were engaged in were defined by tension, name calling, and general lack of communication.

As they become insiders (because of either paid or unpaid activities) within a web of other agencies or community groups or both, they are often critical of ways in which local politics happens. Some of this is a clash in competing ideologies. There are pushes within the HIV-positive community for what several of the women say is to stay "community and client centered." At the same time this viewpoint can compete with women's personal political ambitions, as well as their ability to network and coalition build outside of local community struggles.

A number of the women move back and forth between the desire to work with HIV-positive people to build a larger, more organized, and more visible HIV/AIDS movement in Detroit and Michigan, versus staying locally focused (i.e., in the neighborhood). Over time a few of the women have embraced the criticisms and contradictions; they are sought out and become part of powerful allegiances. And although some of the women often expressed that they did not like the "politics" of a given situation, they still retained a sense of drive and determination about their activities.

Valerie advances the discussion of the dislike and distrust of the political realm. Her comments correspond with other respondents. She works in the same agency that Nicole does—Partnership and Participation in Health Organization. She has a paid position working with people with HIV, and also volunteers her time throughout the greater Detroit area as a resource person on HIV/AIDS. She calls herself an advocate. Her primary focus has been working with HIV-positive people with substance use issues.

> VALERIE: *I have to say I don't like the politics, because it interferes with the issues of my clients. I don't like the politics. Not only does it kind of overwhelm me, but you have to always watch your back. I don't like the dealing with funding sources or dealing with committees. I just don't. I'm more client centered, I like working with the people who are real. I do* [much emphasis]. *I'm in The Engagement Bureau,*[8] *so I do go out and I talk, but it's not about addressing fund-raisers. It's about people, and people who are living with this [disease], and trying to let people know that you can live with this, and you don't have to die. You know. Don't give HIV more power than it has, because you have some control. And so, I want to deal with people, people like me, not all of this . . . Congress. Because someone else can do that.*

Valerie's additional comments illustrate an earlier point about the pitfalls of coalition building. She describes an experience with another agency:

> VALERIE: *I've really had to calm myself down at meetings, which I often get sent to.* [she rolls her eyes and pauses] *You know, as well as I do, what the conditions are for HIV-positive women in this city, let alone the state. Well, last week I had to go to a meeting on how to raise the public awareness about people with HIV in prison. A local council person is concerned about HIV in prison. HIV-rates in prison are soaring. Is he concerned about people, about people with HIV, not in prison?*
> MICHELE: *I did not know.*
> VALERIE: *No, he's not concerned about that! That's a whole other kettle of worms. It's not that I think it's not a good thing . . . Anyway, they want my agency to cosponsor two initiatives with them. It involves money and people. Now it's fine they are doing*

this for people in prison . . . and the public. But you know what is going to happen?
They are going to want to pull myself and other people into this project and it will be a
waste of time. And us here, we're always in the eye of the storm, we won't get anything
in return.

This distrust of the political is also mirrored in the suspicion some of the women have toward other women who are seen as "hooked up" and embedded in local politics. Politics is often perceived as the art of "butt kissing." They were adamant that they did not want to engage in overly accommodating behaviors. One respondent commented, "I've been accommodating half of my life. I want respect and honesty just like the next person. I shouldn't have to beg, plead, or suck up to get the resources this community deserves."

One possible explanation for this sensibility is that women feel they have, in the past, compromised too much to begin to be "nice" *now* in order to get services that they think are their due. They view the political realm as one where there are many constraining social expectations, or as Billy Jean said, "It's hard to speak the truth when everyone is in a business suit, and it's all supposed to be nicey nice." Additionally, some of the reservations respondents expressed could also be attributed to possible unacknowledged fears about what is expected of them in these situations. These fears might be related to worries about their self-presentation and norms about what constitutes "proper" conduct in certain formal political settings. Many women feel uncomfortable by the formality of many aspects of political activity, which involves face-to-face interaction. They are used to working and dealing in a whole different set of social norms. The social norms that govern certain kinds of political work frequently require deference, calmness, ambiguity, and grammatically correct speech; negotiating these required norms are very far removed from the other social environments many of the women have typically inhabited.

Another facet of this phenomenon is the divide between non-HIV-positive people who exert influence in community struggles and HIV-positive people. There are now many women and men who are not HIV-positive who have influence in various HIV-positive networks because of mayoral or state- or governor-appointed positions. Cynthia described one of her encounters in this network. She was interested in working with some of the non-HIV-positive women in positions of power who were helping others attend a conference (on women with HIV) out of state:

CYNTHIA: *No, this is my first time of trying to go with these women, and to listen, get*
the format and the information about it. This lady, like I said, everybody somewhat
likes me, so sometimes it's not a problem. Because sometimes, you start talking to
somebody, they have info that they could help you with, hook you up with something
else, and it goes like a domino effect. And then, but when jealousy or arrogance gets in

there, it's a whole different story. Everybody wants to be a chief and no Indians; you know what I mean?

Cynthia was asked later, since she did not attend the conference, about how her opportunities went with this woman:

> She [another woman, who is not HIV-positive who has influence in the community] has so much input that she knows that I would be a help. She's told me so many times, "Cynthia, I'm going to hook you up with this and hook you up with that," but she never follows through because I'm not a butt-kisser. I am not nobody's follower. And me and her clash with that. She's good people, but . . . to me, if I got some information right here to help you, I don't care if you kiss my butt or not. If it's going to help you to better you so you can be a better person for our community, I would let you know. We don't have to look alike, and dress the same, and talk fancy to be effective. Uh huh. We ain't got to sit at the same table when we go to these conferences and stuff.

Shelly comments on her view of some of the problems working with other non-HIV-positive women in the community:

> SHELLY: Sometimes it's this tight web of people, and you feel like "ain't we all got the same goals?" I'm of the opinion we all have good minds and hearts so give us all a shot. Some women like that whole political angle. It just ain't for me—I like getting stuff done a little differently.

There are also some women who embrace the concept of politics and realize that there will have to be some engagement with a diversity of people and more formal political structures. Nicole is one of those women. Reflecting on far she has come, Nicole stated:

> NICOLE: Girl, do you know what I used to say? I'm not going to be in that political arena, I'm not going to do this and I'm not going to do that. And here I am now, I am part of that. I look at where monies is coming in, what is what. And then my job right now, right here at this agency, I have to know which part of the money is out there for what purpose. Title I is for direct emergencies assistance. Title II is for like primary care and case management. Title IIIB is for primary care, Title IV is for women and children. Title V is for education and training. I have to know these things so that when one of my clients come in, I know where I can best fit them, and their needs and under which, whatever title. That's politics dealing with grants and money. It's politics—knowing who to call when something I need falls through. When people do favors for you . . . that's politics.

As argued in the beginning of the book, women have participated in many varied venues that constitute the political world by definition. How is this possible? It is possible because although the women tend to share a basic distrust of government and politics, they trust *each other* and the networks they, as HIV-positive women, have created together.

Paradoxically, although the women tend to express strong reservations about being involved in "politics," their activities put them squarely in the middle of demands and struggles of who gets to define the "HIV-positive community." Despite this distrust and for some, tactics of psychological distancing, they continue to impact other people and their communities, and often help to shape an agenda of Michigan's policies concerning HIV/AIDS issues. In part the women's resistance to the idea of traditional politics, it is argued, is one of the motivating forces, which facilitates their use of blended and overlapping roles, to be discussed next.

BLENDED AND OVERLAPPING ROLES

The concept of *blended and overlapping roles* is a useful analytical tool in describing the nature and variation in the women's participation. This analysis is drawn from both sociological notions about paid and unpaid community work as comprising "occupational labor" and from social-work concepts of advocacy (Hardcastle, Wenocur, and Powers 1997). Role behavior is an extension of the themes developed in the sociological literature arguing that women community workers (particularly women of color) engage in activities that require a reconceptualization of political practice and social change (see Gilkes 1980, 1988, 1990, 1994; Naples 1991a, 1991b, 1994, 1998). They are often engaged in the types of activities that do not always fall neatly under the traditional definition "of the political." Thus, here in this research their positions are deemed roles to call specific attention to the ways their activities straddle and intersect with labor, community work, and traditional and nontraditional political participation (Gilkes 1988, 1990, 1994; Naples 1994). The argument put forth here posits that because women do not solely identify themselves within a stable category of political identity such as "HIV activist," we can best understand the dynamics (and meanings) of their participation through roles. The term *role* casts a wider analytic net for the purposes of explaining and understanding their pursuits.

There are three roles that I use to describe aspects of the women's formal and informal political activities: *advocates*, *activists*, and *helpers*. Each of these three roles, but particularly the role of advocate, is a role that is embedded in, and that demonstrates the fluidity of community work, paid work, and traditional politics. The word *role* means (1) a character assigned or assumed; (2) a function or part performed especially in a particular operation or process (*Merriam Webster's Eleventh Collegiate Dictionary*). Both meanings connote flexibility, and the term *role* is used intentionally. These terms account for defining women's self-perceptions of their activities. What do roles tell us for this group of stigmatized women? Incorporating these distinctions into conceptualizations of politics helps us to rethink the ways in which women seek to develop and advance their own objectives as well sustain the concept of community.

This concept of blended and overlapping roles demonstrates how the women take up activities that are sometimes beyond the definition of an original role (e.g., an advocate is someone specifically focused on recovery), and extend that role into areas belonging in both the private and the public sphere. The skill and creativity they employ when using these roles help to create and re-create a sense of the HIV-positive community, which is often in the forefront of their concerns.

The second importance of role behavior is that it helps explain their challenges in developing and implementing social change. Each group has a particular set of challenges in defining and maintaining a political space, or a civic space where their interests can take shape. For their recently acknowledged "expertise" in areas related to HIV/AIDS, advocates are valued. However, the women have to negotiate the expectations of committees, task forces, and political projects with their desire to help people with HIV (particularly women with HIV), and stay "client centered." This situation provides continuous challenges to working on behalf of an HIV-positive community. The women who embrace the term "activist" have different types of conflicts. They do not have to straddle the definitions of employment or volunteer work because they are firmly rooted in more established notions of the political. The women who define themselves primarily as helpers have found a way to be active in both the formal and informal realms. Helpers tend to see themselves as bridge people.

An interesting finding arises from apprehension of these roles. Women who call themselves advocates tend to be more focused solely on HIV/AIDS work than either of the other two groups and have more political links across the spectrum. Activists are more diffuse in their interests and have a smaller circle of political contacts; they often find Detroit a difficult city in which to satisfy their larger ambitions; they also tend to be interested in producing cultural products, which challenge and provoke people. Helpers conduct community work that extends into other areas besides HIV/AIDS.

Advocacy

As stated earlier, the majority of the respondents of the deep sample are in some way involved with activities that fall under the broad label of "the advocate" and "advocacy." Early on while conducting this research, the role of the advocate and the concept of advocacy were ignored because they seemed to be laden with therapeutic overtones—and a concept linked solely to substance treatment programs. It was only until later when it was evident that there existed multiple ways in which women used the concept of advocacy for their own purposes, which provided them a set of possibilities to fulfill a larger community mandate; the importance of advocacy theoretically "hit home." A short analytical memo that was written in 1996 describes some of the difficulty (semantically and conceptually) in understanding what advocacy and activism meant to respondents and the researcher.

ANALYTICAL MEMO:
ADVOCACY/ACTIVISM—FALSE DICHOTOMIES?

As I was discovering more about the ways in which women thought of their political activities, I was also confronted with an epistemological dilemma. It centered on my training as a political scientist. Nicole usually calls herself an advocate, not, as she corrected me, an activist. Three women that I have interviewed thus far, however, use the term activist. Many of the others, however, use the term advocate. Some women don't use any words to categorize what they do politically. They often employ the broad term "helping." When trying to understand these terms from a narrative perspective, I think the women communicate something that comes from both an emotional and mental space.

Nicole once said to me: "I love being an activist, or rather an advocate. I really call myself an advocate." At first I didn't understand this distinction, and I always referred to her (and thought of her) as an activist. When I think about advocacy I think of someone speaking on behalf of someone else, a safeguarding of someone, or something. When I would watch Nicole and others give speeches, talk to female juvenile offenders about HIV-risk, and lead marches I would think to myself—"Of course what these women are doing constitutes political activity."

Later, when I thought more deeply about this situation I realized that many of my categories about politics and identity were coming into conflict with her understanding of the activities that she undertook. This is a common occurrence for qualitative researchers (see Gluck and Patai 1991). We can both be right. The work that she undertakes forms a major part of her life, but in many ways she is not defined by it, and essentially activism for me constitutes a more well defined political identity. The activities some of the women undertake are in a way connected with the rest of their lives. I also think that part of this dilemma arises from the often dichotomized ways political scientists and others have conceptualized political activity.

Advocacy at the time *never* meant all the things that could look like "normal politics." The short memo begins to explore some early presumptions I had regarding what constituted political work. What I would add now to the above reflection is that my emphasis on blended and overlapping roles as opposed to strict identity does more to explain the nature of women's participation. We begin with Julianna's experiences as an example of her move from self-advocacy to group advocacy, and later her move to a paid position. Her later narratives illustrate how she uses the place of employment to further her own interests, both professionally and politically.

In the following quote she discusses her early beginnings. She went from being a member of one of Nicole's early support groups to running a group of her own for HIV-positive women, and then being employed.

JULIANNA: *When I stopped paying attention to the others [family members] and started paying attention to me, I changed. I was just like a little sponge; I just started sucking up all this information, because I knew I was behind. But I really didn't miss much, because there's so much misinformation in those years anyway, and I just skipped some stuff. So, then I just started learning this stuff at this incredible speed. You know, because it wasn't like learning, it directed your thinking. So I wanted it all. . . . You know, the more information I got, I got to this point and I was mad as hell. I'm like, the people who run things here in the city about HIV are idiots, and they do not know what they're talking about. At one of my first meetings it was really clear. . . . And they're sitting around trying to make everybody comfortable. And it was obvious, we had nothing to be comfortable about.*

. . . No research had been done on women and HIV. You know, and I was like, oh, man. And they had this life expectancy at the time, I think it was like seven or eight years, or something. People were dying all the time, I was like, oh shit. Then I couldn't get any madder. So I just started fighting back. I just found that if I got the right people to listen to me, and I got more and more information, I started to feel empowered. And then I wanted to make others feel empowered. And then I saw the glitches in the system that didn't seem quite right to me. And I wanted to know why those things were in place that way anyway. And then it just pretty much took off from there. But I was still advocating only for myself.

Julianna advocated for herself for the first three years without any other types of commitments. She then began her own support group out of her house, drawing on some of Nicole's people, but also expanded it to include women from other hospitals and women recently released from prison. She attended several national conferences on women and HIV/AIDS.

She decided to take her current job (Women's Client Manager and Advocate) in part because it allowed her to work with newly diagnosed HIV-positive women. Working in this position, she has administrative and institutional privileges that would not be accessible to her if she was working by herself. On the one hand, many women who find themselves in advocacy positions do so through paid and volunteer efforts. However, this paid employment often increases and augments their ties and commitment to larger political goals on behalf of the community. It routinizes activities for the women. Women such as Julianna move from self-advocacy to paid employment to other types of participation. It also confers respect from other people within HIV-positive communities.

Often in these positions they draw on their larger sense of "being a woman with HIV" to figure out situations when their position does not have clear guidelines about a dilemma involving an HIV-positive person. The employment itself may be a formal extension of advocacy; it may include client services or outreach. It is when there is an unusual situation that the women often draw on their own areas of knowledge and expertise, and sometimes break other agency rules.

Below, she discusses a particular client:

> JULIANNA: *I make sure that any of their needs [newly diagnosed people with HIV] are met. If they have any needs, anything that's going to make their life easier, anything that's government funded that we can do for them, from transportation to "my baby needs a bed," I get them in touch with who can solve the problem.*
>
> *Sometimes it gets real interesting. Like for example, I have an African woman who's here illegally, and is HIV-positive and is pregnant. And speaks only French. So I worked with her yesterday. Just stuff. Because there's all kind of just glitches which will drive me crazy. Now technically, I'm supposed to turn her over to another agency, but you want to know what they'll do? They will probably deport her. I can't have that.*

She went on to discuss how, because of her political contacts she later was able to connect this woman to a number of services, which if done openly would have put her in conflict with her employers. Advocates' emphasis often is on how they can extend themselves. Through her work at the agency, she is able to keep her credibility. Through her work in the community, she has a name as someone who has an "in" at her place.

Two Advocates' Beginnings

NICOLE

Nicole's and Charlene's histories in advocacy work help us understand some of the features of blended and overlapping roles. We first begin with Nicole.

I had heard about Nicole early in my fieldwork, long before I met her. I finally met her by accident through my own contacts. I decided to conduct an oral history with Nicole because of her organizing activities in Detroit. I also wanted to understand how she had become politically active.

She begins her discussion first through her volunteer efforts, which were linked to her recovery efforts. During this time she was trying to understand her own needs regarding her HIV-positive status. She also had come into contact with Charlene, a mover and shaker within the HIV/AIDS community, as well as within substance abuse treatment and prevention services circles.

NICOLE: *When I had about six months clean, the director, she wanted me to start being her assistant. So she paid me an advocacy [volunteer] stipend*[9] *while I was staying in there. And then when I decided to leave the program I had got this other job, a real good job. And I went back up there one day just to visit, and she said would I come and work on the weekend so I said, OK. I went up there and worked that weekend then. The next week she called me up and said, "Do you might want a job on the weekends?" I said, "What you want me to do?" She said, "I want you to come up here and work in Sharon's Place [a treatment center]."*[10]

As argued earlier it is not uncommon for women to combine volunteer activities and extend and overlap them with advocacy. This is an example of the ways in which Nicole was active of her own accord, and how there was an overlap between volunteering, a paid position, and recovery. This continues with Nicole's work at the Department of Health:

OK. When I was about almost to my year clean, I started volunteering at the HIV/AIDS program at the Detroit Health Department.[11] *And so people would call up and like the AIDS program was the 1-800 number, but they always had these problems, and people was always telling me things about different organizations and different things that was going on. And I met some really good friends who I really love over there. Helping those people is what helped me get myself back together. It was like God places you in situations and places where you can really get yourself together. And so anyway, I started to tell the ladies what I thought they should do for themselves. And so they asked me to sit on the Michigan Regional Committee [the board serves areas within southeastern Michigan]. So I sat on there, but I never really said anything. I would wait until after the meeting was over and I would go to them in private and say what I had to say.*

In this following long quote Nicole discusses how she got started specifically in advocacy work. Nicole was invited to attend the AIDS Awareness Workshop because of her extensive volunteer work at the Detroit Department of Health. As discussed in chapter 3 this workshop was held daily in Detroit at the Thirty-sixth District Courthouse. Any man or woman that is arrested for soliciting or carrying drug paraphernalia is required to attend this workshop. She was invited to tell her story as a former sex worker and substance user, and now a woman living with HIV. Nicole enjoyed these interactions, and she quickly made speaking at the workshops a primary activity:

What I used to do, I would give them [women at the workshop] my card about the support group and I would give them my card about substance abuse. I would stand up there and I would tell them a little bit about me. I said all these symptoms that they had I had them. I said don't get them confused with HIV, but still go and get tested. Anytime you have unprotected sex, you need to go and get tested. I said these symptoms that they show right here [points to an imaginary pamphlet], if you have them over seven to ten days, you need to go and get tested. Because the first couple of days could just be you coming down off of getting high. And that's how I got a lot of women to come to support groups. After I told them that I was HIV-positive, they would wait around at the end and they'd come over to me, and say, "I'm HIV-positive." I said, "Girl, you better get your butt off that street." And I told them how crack would make them end up having pneumonia quicker than anything. That's how I talked to them. I got a lot of women in just like that. I remember for our support group, we only started out with two women. It was me, Betty, and Lila to help educate them. And I was the only client there. And I was like, every time I went, I wanted to meet some people. And they said, "Dang, they don't know what was going on." I said, "I'm going out here to get us some for this group." And when they came in that next Thursday, I had about fifteen women at that group. I made sure they had transportation and everything. And they were so pleased they just sat back and let me continue. They had never seen anyone be so "aggressive." That's what they called me.

This passage describes how Nicole clearly casts herself in a heroic as well as determined role in trying to get women into support groups. From this determined start in gathering women in the community, she slowly became involved in other types of activities that intersected with the traditional political realm. This passage also suggests resourcefulness and confidence from these experiences, that one experience was meaningful and led to others. And finally, this incident represents the first step in the process of becoming politically active. She identifies with her own situation and also identifies with other women in similar circumstances; she makes connections.

She surprised and surpassed their expectations at the treatment center. She drew on the role of advocacy, but also began to move away from that as a norm by involving herself in other projects. She led retreats for women with HIV/AIDS. This was not something commonly done in the late eighties or early nineties. She also drew on unusual contacts, soliciting her old drug haunts, and other arenas where she knew women were vulnerable to HIV/AIDS infection. When asked about this direct and unusual approach she said:

Girl, those were the very dark days. I endangered myself sometimes because I kept going to places where I knew women used [crack cocaine]. It really tested my recovery efforts and my faith. But I just kept going because no one was going to really go to those places. People give out condoms and everything, but you know you have to go the source where women are at.

It was many of these incidents that helped to suggest to Nicole that she could make a difference sharing her knowledge with other HIV-positive women in her community. We now turn to an examination of one of her first big political projects.

Detroit's stigmatized women have worked against a very turbulent and punitive political backdrop concerning crime, women and substance abuse, and HIV. Pregnant addicted mothers have become the focus of a moral crisis, and in many states have faced various types of punitive legislation (Chavkin 1991; Paltrow 1990; Roberts 1991). Many have commented on the often racist and classist motivations of legislators (see generally Roberts 1991; Young 1994). One of Nicole's projects was to get a petition submitted in protest of a bill that was debated in the Michigan legislature in 1995. The bill mandated that all pregnant women be tested for HIV/AIDS. A congressman proposed this as the only way the state could get Ryan White money for programs and research that deal with HIV/AIDS. In this passage, Nicole connects how women substance users tend to be targeted, and the overall consequences of stigmatizing women:

> NICOLE: *I already have people signed it [the petition protesting the bill] because I feel like it's wrong because a lot of women would not go to the doctor, they already don't want to go to the doctor. They're substance users and they're embarrassed. And then to make women go get tested and if they are positive, make them be on AZT [medication which helps to prevent HIV antibodies that affect the fetus], I feel it's wrong. A violation of our Constitution. The women did not get HIV-positive by themselves, what about the men? So if you're going to mandate anybody to get tested, you should mandate everybody to get tested. But that would still be a violation.*

She continued her analysis about the problems with such proposed legislation:

> *I thought about this. They [congressmen] are not going to have their wives going to get tested for HIV when their wives get pregnant. So why would they want to do that to the low-income women? That's where I see a line of hypocrisy.*

Mandatory testing is a controversial issue and was widely debated in many states during the 1990s. Mandatory testing of pregnant women tends to reinforce the idea that women are the morally culpable ones regarding the spread of HIV/AIDS and transmission to children. It also suggests they should shoulder the majority of social responsibility. Mandatory testing would tend to disproportionately affect lower income women accessing state funded programs. Nicole organized and gathered petitions from her own efforts, not drawing on resources of her employed situation. She organized around making the public aware of the factors that lead women to become HIV-positive. Nicole was able to mobilize other interests to support her beliefs, including local Detroit women's groups and the local ACLU. They helped make this legislation appear as a combination of violation of privacy and a gender discrimination issue. State representatives also took a keen interest in the mobilization that Nicole was able to direct. She devoted an enormous amount of time and energy to this issue.

The result was a compromise between all sides. If through various efforts Michigan did not specifically reduce the rates of HIV/AIDS perinatal transmission within five years, then the legislature could decide to attach a requirement of mandatory testing of pregnant women to Ryan White federal funding. Pragmatically oriented and concerned about both women and children who have HIV, Nicole, when asked about this compromise, responded:

> But in five years we have our time to do our work, and if we don't then we should have it on there. We should be doing something out there so the community will be thanking us, and won't have to worry about their babies being infected. You know what I'm saying? Five years is a long time to be working on something so women don't be infected and their babies don't be infected.

Her concern for stigmatized women stems from her connections with other women and her life experience. On a daily basis, Nicole works with women that are having problems with their primary care providers, women who are in denial about their HIV-positive status, and women who have no familial or other support systems in dealing with the challenges of having the HIV/AIDS virus. In the following quote, Nicole demonstrates an understanding of the severity of HIV/AIDS stigma for women. This quote comes from one of the early interviews:

> I just want to be able to say what I have to say on behalf of the community and behalf of people who are HIV-positive. Especially for women, because a lot of women are still sitting in the house, they're isolated, they're being caregivers, they can't stand up and say they're HIV-positive because they got kids and they don't want their children to be embarrassed or anything like that. They don't want their kids to have to go through that. Either they will look at their mother like she was a crack head or a prostitute, something like that. And they won't look at it like the man gave it to the women and stuff. A lot of women are still in denial about it. They're ashamed, they hurt. All of the above. Somebody got to stand up for them. I don't have nothing to be ashamed of. I'm not embarrassed, my family is sticking by me 100. And so I feel like I'm good going out there talking on their behalf. I try to encourage more women with children to stand up. If they won't stand up, I'm going to have them sign petitions like this. I tell them the only way that society will start listening to us is the women stand up more, come out more in numbers. I say, "How can I stand up and talk about your problem if you won't come and stand up and talk about your problems?"

CHARLENE

Charlene as an advocate has been able to advance critiques of two things: (1) the inadequacies of certain programs that purport to serve people with the HIV virus, but in her opinion do little except collect Medicaid and other forms of insurance and (2) the importance of literacy and self-education projects for former substance users and the wider HIV-positive community. These ideas expressed within traditional advocacy/employment roles have caused her to be fired and face substantial criticism. Although the community supports her work (and has often rallied behind her) and although she has truly enjoyed her work, facing these challenges has taken an emotional toll. She discussed advocacy:

CHARLENE: *I don't even know the difference between an advocate and activist. I don't care, I always say an advocate. Yeah. I guess I would say advocate, because I see a lot of things going on and I must do something about that, wherever it takes me. Whatever that entails for my job and outside of it. Especially dealing with the families. A lot of families are not accepting of people with HIV. These is your kids, I don't care what they have. I mean, this family I know told me [her client], "Look, we don't care what you got and what you did. Do me one favor, don't go get high. That's all we ask you." If more families were like that, understanding, wanting to become educated, it would be okay*

. . . See, we ain't got no sense of what's happening because half of us can't read, and they ain't going to take you seriously if you can't read. They don't have education. They don't understand what you're talking about. They don't understand what the doctor tells them or gives them. The doctor don't tell them nothing about medication, you know. And I tell people, when you go to the doctor, ask them this, there's an A, B, C, D. Ask them about medication they're going to put you on, what it's going to do, what type of side effects it have, what's going on with your body. . . .

She has organized people in the community to volunteer their time for reading and tutoring at the agency where she works. She discusses her earlier work, how she decided to specialize in substance abuse issues, and helping Nicole:

I ran support groups. I went to a lot of different support groups. I got Nicole. I helped her really get started. I went into substance abuse, I went on and got certified, and I'm an HIV/AIDS instructor. And when she came in, I decided to help her.

I told her, "Go for what you know." You're good in the HIV and AIDS, which I'm not going to say that I'm not, I just didn't get off into it the way she did because I've been in substance abuse since 1987. And you know, that's the kind of work I've been doing, so when I need information from her, I get it, and when she need it from me, I can give it to her, and it worked like that, instead of, you know, us hoarding everything. She's good at it, you know what I'm saying? And I know I'm good at substance abuse.

Over several interviews, Charlene discussed how difficult it is for new people in the HIV/AIDS community (especially substance users) to identify with the ability to live free from drugs and create a healthy lifestyle. Charlene, among others, provides an example of positive things to do in the community.

Regardless of how they look at me, and how well I'm doing, they're saying that's Charlene. But they still want to continue to get high. They think they're not ready to deal with the issues. When it's basically left up to them in the treatment center, they do,

I guess they do what they can do. And I guess that's all that is. I guess it's basically left up to them, but they need more people that's willing to help them. They help them with houses and all this type of stuff. But yeah, but what about the continuous counseling behind that? Don't leave them hanging. Because as soon as the situation arises, they're going to run out, and they're going to get high. So they don't have that continuous support, and then their insurance is all messed up, so we're losing.

I was able to observe the many long hours Charlene committed to working with clients. She is one of the few women who talked a lot about over-arching concerns with this population.[12]

After getting an overall picture of the beginnings of some advocates, let us turn to how women negotiate their job and community sensibilities.

I WON'T SELL MY SOUL: ACROSS THE DIMENSIONS
OF ADVOCACY—PAID AND UNPAID WORK

Women who take paid positions do so with the intention of furthering their goals of HIV/AIDS related work. This presents challenges, both internal and external. Advocates face specific challenges: there is the price of inclusion (of being the token "HIV person") and the tension about deciding where the ever-shifting set of community boundaries lie. On the one hand, advocacy work often offers them the stability of a paid position. Women, however, maintain role boundaries by being willing to walk away from paid positions in their advocacy work. This willingness to walk away helps them to maintain their focus and their dignity around issues that are important to them. In the following discussion, Julianna decided to tell me about the local politics of the HIV-positive community, which she is often dragged into:

JULIANNA: *I don't care. I really don't. And it's interesting to see them come from just all these different angles, you know, and try to suck me into this mire that they've created. And you know, I don't care. I'm on a real natural high. I don't care. I have my work here and outside, I'm happy with this job, you know, but I'm not going to sell my soul for it.*

She reflects on other opportunities for employment in these areas and their potential pitfalls:

I'm going to get what I can out of this. . . . I have no idea how I could be doing this at all. I never even dreamed it. But I will be employable in any of these factions. Even in the health department. And then wait, after I get this job, right, the health department calls [and offers her a position]. They have got to be crazy. Like I would work for them. There is no way I could work for them.[13]

I was not here a year, now you want me, right? And I had not been on the job long enough to decide whether, you know, this was my little niche. Should I go there? I was like, man, it always comes like that. And if anyone thinks that when I come over there it's going to be easy for them. . . . Not a chance. I have a vision, which is outside some of these people's parameters.

Julianna illustrates in the above passage what other women have discussed. Just because they have opted to have a paid position committed to working for the HIV-positive community does not mean that they have sole allegiance to an institution. For Charlene the experiences of the volunteer position, advocacy positions, and then her new position, which combines advocacy related work, for her was a source of stability and pride. Her advocacy-type work was the first time she had a legitimate job.

CHARLENE: *I had never lived by myself, never worked, never went to school, never did nothing, never paid a bill. I didn't have to pay bills. All right, now how do you do this? How do you pay bills? And I said, yeah, that makes sense. If you want something, go put it in layaway, yeah that makes sense. I say, how do you do that? Go put it in layaway. You know what I'm saying? So, it's stuff like that. You have to ask, you have to find somebody that's willing to help you and not use you. And that's what I did.*

Yeah, it's hard. I mean, none of this stuff happened overnight. . . . I know that I can get out there and work for it. . . . Anything I want, I had to learn that.

I have to get out there and get, because nothing comes free no more. See, it came free when I was out there, because I was taking it. Don't nothing come free no more. That's what you got to learn. And it's OK to work eight hours a day, even though I don't, I work six hours. . . . Everything I buy is not brand new. But it's mine. You know what I'm saying? I tell people you can do it, but don't live above your means. And you have to learn how to not live above your means. And I work six hours a day, three days a week, and I can pay my rent, and I can pay every bill I created, for the first time in my life.

Despite the overall goodwill feelings many of the advocates have about their positions, they are not willing to compromise their principles. It is a repeated theme among the advocates that even though they have a paid position, that does not mean they are at the disposal of others' agendas. This sense of allegiance to a larger community as well as being in a "human service worker" position corroborates Naples's understanding of the challenges of the community worker:

The job of the indigenous community worker is not "9 to 5." Most community workers did not view their jobs merely as a source of income. Their commitment to their communities contributed to a blurring of lines between their paid responsibilities and their unpaid activities. (Naples 1991a, 321)

As women gain more of a sense of efficacy regarding their advocacy and become people who are respected and confided in, their understanding of what is possible changes. Nicole has sharpened her sense of what is possible for women now that she's an "insider" in Detroit's women and AIDS policy circles. She says, "I see a lot of waste. They should have never have let me get on the inside, because I see too much waste." Nicole has voiced her own critical assessments of community committees and task forces set up for HIV/AIDS intervention and prevention:

And then, as I started growing up more, I started reading more, learning more. I said this ain't right. I'm going to say something about it.

Nicole was appointed to a main advisory committee on women and HIV, and had to work with experts and health professionals in the field who she feels are often not as devoted to the issues as she is:

NICOLE: *I'm like everybody's always wanting to do this job with HIV and AIDS, but sometimes I wonder where people's hearts really are because when HIV and AIDS came out especially now, they see a lot of money. They see dollar signs, and they don't see feelings anymore. They always talk about money this, money that. They're always talking about data this, data that. What about the real people? What about the needs of the people? And they said they try to meet the needs, but they're not.*

During another interview Nicole explored similar themes:

Even though I got a Title I job. A lot of times people won't say nothing because that's where they're getting their bread and butter from. But to me, it don't matter because I'm going to get a job anyway. I can go back out and get a private-duty nursing job.

Charlene recounted an incident where principles were tested that resulted in her leaving a position:

CHARLENE: *Yeah, I use to work at the walk-in clinic downtown as an advocate. I stayed there only eleven months, they fired me because of my mouth.*
MICHELE: *What do you mean?*
CHARLENE: *Because I tell you what I feel, and I don't care what you think about it . . . the people running the clinic didn't appreciate that. I was arguing about getting more services, they didn't want to write grants or do nothing.*
MICHELE: *Was that your job?*
CHARLENE: *Nope. But, everybody was in the wrong. Everybody was in the wrong. We kept referring people to a residential program which let people stay there supposedly to help them with HIV. Well the state has a limit on how much they'll spend on those programs, so after six, nine months, the people are back on the streets or even worse. We needed better transitional programs at the clinic, and I got tired of referring people to these programs to see them bounce right damn back in my lap.*

They told me I was out of order, and that I didn't know what I was talking about I said, "Keep your job." Then I went over to LifeHelp[14] and I've been there since 1991. I enjoy counseling and advocacy, I like what I do. I've helped a lot of people, I've seen a lot of people fail. I've seen a lot of them die.

Women often distinguish their activities from others on the basis of non-HIV-positive status or positive status. They tend to view themselves as more knowledgeable than their peers, and especially more committed than many of the other people in the organization. Nicole is a senior case manager and has a heavy caseload at any given time. She sees only women who are HIV-positive, some with histories of substance use.

> NICOLE: *Right now I got about forty clients every month. I have had almost a hundred. But when the case manager left the program, a lot of clients on there were like what you call delinquent, and that was because we didn't do, we hadn't done a lot of proper monitoring and stuff, and so when I became the case manager here, I do what really was supposed to be done. And my boss thought the case management was okay like it was. But they just hired somebody in because they wanted to get the money.*
>
> *But now I can say case management is really together. I try to provide services for clients within two days, try to get them in [to see] the doctor. If they're newly diagnosed, within five to ten days after diagnosis so they can go ahead on to the doctor so they won't have to worry, because that's one of the number one worries was, "Should I take medication, should I do this." "Well, really, just go to the doctor and talk to the doctor just like you're talking to me." You know.*

So, before moving on to discuss other aspects of advocacy work, it is important to reiterate that although the women are quite proud of their jobs and work they do, they do not feel that they should sacrifice their voice or sense of integrity. They bring a double-edged consciousness about their work.

ADVOCACY OUTSIDE AN AGENCY OR ORGANIZATION

We move on to the experiences of Constance. Constance has undertaken advocacy work for the past two years. Her advocacy is unconnected to an agency or institution. Her narrative illustrates other routes into advocacy, and that advocacy is as much a position which can be "socially bestowed" onto you by others, as well as claimed by one's self. Constance's foundation of advocacy grows out of her prior professional status as a registered nurse.

Constance is a person who has experienced many of the push-pull factors that make up advocacy work. The second time that I met with Constance, she was wearing a silk scarf with a fuchsia and black abstract print. She was eager to tell me of her struggles in dealing with HIV/AIDS issues and medical and support group concerns. Her focus for the last year and a half has been improving medical service providers' attitudes toward women with HIV and seeing better distribution and use of resources in city- and state-funded HIV/AIDS support groups. She believes she is still in the skills-building stage of advocacy work.

When I first talked with Constance about these concerns, Constance was keenly aware of some of ways in which there were differences between how different ethnic groups got treated within the HIV/AIDS outreach arena. We talked at length about local funding for support groups. At the time she was going to a group sponsored by Hispanic Community Support (HCS).[15] Before that she traveled farther out to attend predominately white support groups.[16] There have been many tensions with the staff and clients at HCS. Constance had never really considered any advocacy work. However, she began to take actions on behalf of herself and her group. Her agitation revolved around trying to get more resources for the groups, diversify the events, and make better use of the existing resources. Now Constance's concern is in this instance primarily personal, but also stems from her convictions that people with HIV/AIDS are treated poorly by various agencies. She goes on to explain the arrangement of how these groups work. In doing so she explains how some of the support groups, sponsored by city agencies, operate:

CONSTANCE: *Yeah. these HIV-positive groups [pauses and shakes her head]. There are all kinds of groups now that you can go to. And you know, the person at an agency sends a fax to another agency, a fax that says, "We would like for you to join us on Friday evening, we're having a potluck." And you [a facilitator] go back and tell the people of the group, you know, well, this agency would like to have you over. Would you like to come? You know, or something like that. Now I've seen we got a lot of invitations, from different places doing different things. And I mentioned some of them and the facilitator just told me disregard it. Why can't you take [the] HCS van and say, well, OK, we've been invited out, we're going to go and you know, network with them. That's what it's supposed to be like. You know. This is the whole southeastern Michigan thing, and we're all funded. These agencies are all funded, mostly under the Ryan White title act. And they're supposed to work together. But then when you get a facilitator that's not interested, you know, and will not return the person's call, and the example I'm telling you, it's a fact that the facilitator did not return the call, because Annette [from another agency] called me. I called her back, and she says, "Well, Constance, do you think that I should still send her a fax?" I said, "I would do that, too." The facilitator never acknowledged it, never said anything. She never came to the group and asked, "Would you like to go out that evening, having a potluck and games and fun?" Social night, you know. Never. I think because she's just not interested. To her it's just a job, and whatever she has planned, you know. "OK, well, I'll take you guys to Boston Chicken to eat." But she will not call all these people who are signing their names all the time, you understand what I'm saying? No, you know. And you know when we go down there to HCS, she will call lots of people, so it would look like she's got a lot of people [on the sheet which gets sent to the state] to impress them.*

And you know, I get so disgusted going to these groups, and as soon as you get there they want you to sign your name. Sign your name so they can turn it in, so they [the agency] can continue to be funded. And it's not fair that people are capitalizing on people with HIV and AIDS.

And half of the people will not come when they get their SSI, or whatever on the first of the month. They're busy doing their thing, paying bills, or if they're drug addicts they got money, and they don't come until like they're hungry, they need a food box or whatever. . . . And these kinds of things frustrate me, you know. And so we had a meeting, oh, I think, maybe last month. And I really got on her about this. And she says, "Well, you can feel free to speak to my supervisor. I have a new supervisor, and she seems to be really on the ball." But you know, I haven't talked to her yet, and everything.

Constance went on to discuss other ways in which the women of the group were disrespected, including poor planning of topics, waiting for hours for transportation to meetings, and general stagnation. Below she elaborated on other problems:

And at the support group . . . which is supposed to be for all, they're really for their nationality. They're for Hispanics. But in order to be up under the [federal] umbrella, they have to bring in blacks. You see what I'm saying? They have to bring in blacks. So naturally, they get, they have a Black group set up. And this black group is allowed X amount of money to plan events, bring in speakers, or we go on a couple of little trips, or whatever. But then you find out that the person who's getting the money goes to her home, fixes the food, and brings it to the group you know what I'm saying? People with HIV and AIDS can't eat certain things [emphatically].

. . . Like in my case, I can't eat spicy spaghetti, which is going to give me diarrhea, [or] soupy tuna macaroni salad. You know. And I think, you know, if they're going to give them money, well they should allocate their resources better, say for instance, in Lynn's group [another facilitator]; I don't think it's fair for her to go home and cook a meal. She's not a licensed dietitian. She does not know what the people in the group want. We have to drive by her house, pick up a meal and then go serve it. That's not fair. Because like I spoke to her, and then wrote a letter to her supervisor, and I'm like, you know, you can buy two chickens and cut them up and fry them. And buy lettuce and tomato or prepackaged salad. That does not equal out to what they're giving you. So what's happening with the other money? Why can't this other money be put over into a pool, and we use it to go out or to the show, or whatever, you know. And we have these groups and we don't do anything. And then I was saying, well why don't we network out to other groups? You know. And then I sent her a letter based on my comments . . . what I'm telling you today.

The above highlights structural problems with agencies (state and federally funded) running support services in Detroit; these are often issues that have not been examined as important factors in HIV-positive women's overall support systems. Racial and ethnic issues may get played out differently in other large metropolitan areas. Constance's insights suggest that there is the assumption among some who work with HIV-positive people that women with HIV will *take* what they can get.

Upon interviewing her some time later, she had begun to see herself differently, and indeed the women of her group and others began to inquire if she wanted to be an advocate—meaning taking part in seminars, trainings, speaking opportunities, and the like. She was getting a reputation for being someone who knew how to speak to authorities and was shrewd.[17] Soon, women in the community started treating her like someone who already was an advocate.

Moreover, because of her professional status as a former registered nurse, many women, in particular, approached her for advice or when they were having problems with their medical providers. By this time, her focus had shifted to medical providers and treatment of HIV-positive patients, a minor theme in previous interviews. In discussing her concerns, she highlighted how she has struggled in her own personal life with doctors who do not listen, who are rude and insensitive, and who are not supportive of her asking questions. When interviewed she was having second thoughts about being on the variety of medications suggested. Although she had a female doctor, whom she thought she would be able to "bond" with, she has been unhappy with her treatment:

> But I'm really angry with myself, because I wouldn't have took this medication, but I took it because of I didn't want to hear her mouth. She tries to argue me down. I'm not satisfied with this doctor. So many people aren't. And then the thing of it is, there's no communication between the patient and the person. It's like the doctors are in a hurry, hurry, hurry, hurry. I don't care if you're going to a fire, they're always in a hurry. And see with this disease you can't be under a lot of stress, because it messes your chemistry up. You know, it stresses you out.

During an interview, she discussed two incidences as a patient which left her feeling angry and that her dignity and respect had been slighted. The first incident involved a physician's assistant calling Constance's home asking for personal information over the phone. The assistant also disclosed her status, and other very personal information was left on Constance's answering machine. She was extremely upset by this incident, citing the fact that she has a grandson who could have overheard that information, and that she deserves privacy like other patients.

At this time during the interview she also discussed her treatment by another doctor, which reaffirmed her notions that people with HIV/AIDS have little privacy and people generally tend to show them a lack of respect. Constance filed a grievance at the hospital after this incident. She was going for an examination and a special treatment for her legs. Notice how in this passage, while describing her response, she also segues into a discussion of how other women have called her for support and guidance:

> I couldn't feel it. He went through the muscle and everything [with a needle], but then again I've been having more problems with my legs. I was dressed in a gown. And I was up on the bed, and he was doing it. So in comes another intern. And I said, "Why are you here? Why are you in my room?" Oh this is Dr. So and So. I said, "But

regardless, you're here and you're watching, and so forth and everything." Then come to find out, the doctor who did it, he was just in his fourth year, this was going to be his last year. I said, "They refer us to these people, they're interns. They don't be the top specialist and stuff. Everybody gets to practice on somebody like me like a guinea pig." And I'm very upset about that. And by me being in the medical field, they really get upset with me when I tell them. But I'm like, no. And people call me, a lot of women from support groups, "What do you think I should do?" And I tell them. They have got to take a step and make doctors slow down and tell them something. But the ladies call me when they don't like something with the nurses or the doctors. I get at least one phone call a week. But see, when you question doctors, or people, they think you're being smart. But it's just the point. It's your body, you know.

After these incidents she went to an out of state conference where her networking invested her with a sense of hope and faith in herself and, also suggested she could help others:

It was really, really great. Soooo much information about what they're doing for the people with HIV. Social security, new medications that they have, what works best with another controlled substance. They went down the line to tell you what the medication does. I enjoyed it so much. It really affected me. There's so much to learn and share with people.

I asked, Were there men?

Right, men and women. So we're having another one this coming March. I mean we had over fifty something people. Way over fifty. And it was really nice. We stayed just the one night, but this time we're going to try and stay a weekend, Friday, Saturday and Sunday. And it's supposed to be more informative, because they have people that come out, they have doctors, they have people from California to let you know what's going on, what to expect. The doctors out there are more friendly and able not to talk down to us, like folks here in Detroit.

After this experience, she commented on some of the actions she had taken thus far:

Oh, I always enjoyed nursing. You know, that's rewarding and everything. So, I really wanted to do a little advocacy work, you know. Maybe, go into the schools or into the prisons and talk about HIV, and get better at dealing with the doctors. You know, keeping a check on them . . . like checks and balances. So, I went to some workshops on different types of subjects, here and there around Detroit.

As Constance began talking about what types of classes she went to on HIV/AIDS issues, she also implicitly discussed her distrust of government and also talked about the political world in relation to HIV-positive people:

Government. It was mostly through the government, too. And they pay you for going to the classes, and all this and stuff, and everything. But everything is done through the government. All this money they got floating around. All this money. And it's some power thing, it's a money. It's a money thing. I went to a women's luncheon down at the ——— Hotel last month. And it was, oh, I don't know, over thousand women that were there. And they had a lot of named [famous] people,

. . . all these people were here, and we went, our HIV group went; I wanted them to go and got everything together. It was so nice, and they were talking about the money and the funds that they get and what they're doing. I met a lot of people there. But after that I had people call me about being an advocate. They don't have this, they don't have a place to stay, they have this or that set of problems. And they'll tell them, we don't have the money, and you just got to go. So there's nowhere for them to turn. Then when they go into like into a homeless shelter or something like that it's really bad. You know, it's really bad. So I talk with them and tell them what I know, and sometimes we get together and I go over some ideas about doctors, et cetera. So in a way, I feel sort of fortunate, and in a way I don't.

She knows many of the people who treat her and encourage her under the rubric of "the advocate," yet she is still suspicious of some of the institutional power it entails. After she had taken some state-funded workshops on advocacy, she had mixed things to say:

They teach you some things, like common sense really. But I already knew how to do some the things they said. It was more informational, but it still doesn't solve all this stuff with the doctors that I told you about before. People just come find me when they need to find me. I'm glad I got to learn a few new things. I guess advocacy is my second nature, really.

I figure while I'm here, and I'm into all these things and working with them, I'm going to try and make a difference. But it's hard most of the time, it's hard.

When I last saw Constance she had just come back from a weeklong conference on women and HIV held in California. She was entirely enthusiastic about the women she met and what she was able to give information on the state of Michigan:

My phone is ringing off the hook. I sure can't put up my feet to rest. Me and this other woman from the support group are going to try to write a small grant. I have to start from square one, but it's okay. We left that support group and are just working on some other things together.

Constance's slow and steady move into advocacy work, outside of institutional support (except for classes), parallels other women's involvement. It begins often in the realm of the self or personal before moving out to affect others. Georgia had this to say a few years before she became involved in other forms of advocacy:

I don't know. It's something I always wanted to do. I wanted to be a person that worked with people, OK. I wanted to be a person to be able to give information. Because I soak in a lot, you know what I'm saying. They're trying to make me be an advocator [sic], now I can. I don't want to be. I want to keep on practicing on my computer, learn how to work that real good. And I want to learn how to do things better, you know what I'm saying. I like words and systems.

Georgia, along with Constance, is one of the few women who consider themselves advocates who do not primarily work out of an HIV/AIDS program, state-run agency, or drug rehabilitation program. Her own self-definition wavers between that of an advocate and a helper. She originally resisted becoming an advocate, though she took advantage of some state funding for HIV-positive people to develop certain life/advocacy skills. Georgia has worked extensively with one community center on the west side of Detroit in developing an arts program geared toward HIV-positive and recovering women. She has developed her writing and speaking skills, and is often asked to give readings of her poems. Georgia has also worked as part of a city coalition that sponsors HIV workshops in the public schools, again using arts as a way to break down people's inhibitions. She believes that advocacy work can be undertaken on many different fronts.

In her helping role, Georgia performs many tasks for other advocates. She has superb organizational and math skills and is often called upon as a treasurer for small, independently run collectives of HIV-positive women. She also possesses significant computer skills and on various occasions has helped Daria, for example, create a database for those who received her newsletter on sexual trauma and HIV-positive women (to be discussed in the activist section).

Helpers

The category of helpers is one that refers to the more generalized and harder to classify group of women who work within the general HIV/AIDS frame. They do not refer to themselves as advocates (though some have in the past embraced aspects of that role), and definitely not as activists. They often refer to the work they do as supporting others, "being there," "doing what it takes," and as *helping*. These activities take the form of volunteer work and projects that they join in on with other women. Most often they help other women, such as advocates, with setting up a support group, sending out a mass mailing for an upcoming event, calling people, taking care of the kids so that women can attend important events. These are also women who will fix food at the gatherings. Additionally, they primarily do work with young people, informally or formally. They are not connected to other agencies or institutions. Women in the community who are active as advocates and activists tend to serve as important contacts for these women. Helpers are more religiously focused than the other two groups.

Although, it is not a specific occupational role, their work or helping is very important to their self-definition and earns respect from their peers for their level of involvement. They also build bridges between advocates and activists because they are more flexible in pursing their goals.

THE RELIGIOUS SPHERE

In most treatment programs, one of the most effective therapeutic practices is an appeal to a higher authority for help and guidance. Although the appeal to religious ideologies was not a part of every treatment program where research was conducted, nor were all the women interested, it was a predominant influence throughout the treatment process. Historically, African American women have exerted power and influence through various churches (see in relation to civil rights Giddings 1984). Indeed, the history of participation for many women is connected to religious organizations (see Cott 1987). Until recently scholars have overlooked, especially for minority women, the ways in which authority in the church and expressions of religiosity is a vehicle for social status.

Although several women made reference to their faith or how the power of their worship helped with their ability to abstain for drugs, they often kept personal beliefs outside of their political involvement. Cynthia's interest and ability within the sphere of HIV/AIDS work stems from her ability to posit herself as a spiritual authority figure within in a community of other women. Cynthia had an early interest in advocacy and went to several of Nicole's groups:

> CYNTHIA: *She's really a good person. And I started and kept going to the meetings there, and going to other women's meetings. Nicole's got kind of boring. Wasn't getting nothing out of it, it was just like a place to eat and meet women, and I was like, I needed more than that. And plus I had very good medical care, all my doctors were excellent, at that time. I was also getting to a point that anything you want to give me or talk to me about regarding HIV, I'm interested. So I would take everything, I was just starting to get notes on my own. I got a whole cabinet here* [points] *full of stuff on AIDS and HIV. One day I'm hopefully going to be an advocate for people with HIV and AIDS.*

At the same time that Cynthia expressed interest in advocacy, she also discussed her relationship to God, and a desire to be pointed into work that was meaningful by a higher standard:

> *See, that's where it gets to the kind of confusing part. I know God has a purpose for me. . . . I really want to be with my family and stuff, but I really want to be able to give to God, too. So it's like, I'm praying God don't be disappointed. But I really want to be of service.*

Cynthia's advocacy work never happened. Instead, she followed her own leanings and dealt with the spiritual and religious aspects of women struggling with drug addition and HIV. In beginning to discuss her activities in relation with HIV, she told a narrative about her interaction with another young woman who was just recovering from heroin withdrawal.

An outpatient treatment program sponsored the retreat for one of the groups Cynthia occasionally attended. The woman was an associate of someone else and new to the recovery process; all the women, including Cynthia, were going on a retreat, or a social. This is the first time that Cynthia ever tried to use her spiritual gifts in a direct way. Cynthia has used spirituality as part of her identity that allows her to be bold, center stage, and take charge. Her "public voice" is developed through her understanding of her mission and God's work. Cynthia was upset that the other women at the retreat gave the woman a holier-than-thou attitude regarding former drug use:

> *"Oh, I used to do this." When you say, "I used to do this," when you're talking to somebody who's just been clean for three days off of heroin, her stomach is doing flips and everything. She don't need to hear that. She needs somebody to hold her, pray with her, and just be there for her. That was not happening. So, I got, I'm a very sensitive person. So, I went to her. I prayed about it. Ironically, because I said, "Lord, make a way that I could come help this lady."*
>
> *Yeah, so I'm praying to God. I couldn't even eat all my food and stuff, I just stopped doing what I was doing. Everybody left, I was the last person out of the kitchen and everything. And when I came outside, she was on the porch. OK, I'll just start walking. I didn't mind the walk . But when I looked over, she was sitting out there smoking a cigarette. Somebody said something to me, was making some kind of crack to me about prayer. I said, "Well, I'll pray for anybody. Wherever I'm at, I'm not ashamed of God." So she's like, "Come over here, pray for me." And there was a door opened. So when I went over there, I just didn't jump in and pray with her, I was talking to her and I told her, "You know, God loves you, you are special." And I was like, what happened? I said, "You're the one that was clean for three days?" And she said, yeah, and I said, OK. I said, "You know, you've been very, very strong in doing this. How do you do it?" She said, "I'm going through this sickness, I feel terrible." She said, "I just want you to pray with me."*

She went on to discuss her interactions with the woman. From this point on, other people asked if Cynthia would help out speaking at some events, about faith and HIV/AIDS issues. Cynthia is a speaker who is very much in demand. When she is not speaking, she is running errands for other women in the support groups and sharing information. But she does not call herself an advocate. When asked why, she replied:

> *All of this [about her activities] was unexpected. Miss Crenthall [an organizer] called me, and whenever Miss Crenthall calls me to go with her to do something, to be a spokesperson, or be on the panel, I go, because I know, she's good people and she's not going to lead me wrong. I help people get to where they need to be. I don't have to have a fancy title or anything. Just even introduce me. That's all they got to do. Just introduce me. I can do the rest. God and me can do the rest.*

Cynthia enjoys talking with young people. She does not discuss religious matters with them, but focuses on HIV/AIDS prevention and abstinence from drugs. Even though she does not discuss God with them, her perception of her abilities during the event is related to God. She recounted a particularly moving experience in her work with young people:

Yeah, and it was all black girls, you know, students and stuff, and I was just overwhelmed. And they listened to my story, and it wasn't like, I'd been in front of an audience and everybody's doing one of these numbers [makes gestures that she's yawning], and, but these girls, there was about thirty of them, they were so into it, and then the Lord and the Holy Spirit was in it too, and it touched a lot of their hearts. A couple of them was crying. Not for sadness, but I really believe from, they acted like they wept with me through the whole thing, and it's like they seen the Jesus and joy and the power of God now in working through me, and it was just overwhelming. And I wish my daughter was there. I knew I was helping them.

Cynthia has worked with various black churches in the area of Detroit, prompting them to coordinate and develop more services for people with HIV, and has challenged discriminatory attitudes on the part of religious leaders. She's faced enormous resistance, though she has also had some breakthroughs:

They hardly want to talk about how drugs got a hold of our communities. I work with them, and I ask God to let them see me for me, a servant of his words. One project though gave me hope. I worked on it with another sister. We had two Sundays set aside for four churches to have their congregation come in and discuss HIV/AIDS with people that's got it. We got a good turnout. You have to just try new and different things. I also helped out with the youth discussion part. It was a big success.

Due to Cynthia's respect within several circles of African American churches she has been asked to lend her time to other issues outside of HIV/AIDS, including the fight for adequate low-income housing throughout the city and against police brutality. I asked her to comment on these newer developments:

Why not is what I said to myself? Why not? I am a full human being and I do care about what is happening with people finding decent, safe places to live. I don't want to take too much time away from HIV/AIDS thing because that is what I love to do. But, I also can't say no to a minister who asks me to show up at a rally or a meeting with some high level officials, now can I? Somehow, I'm gonna find a way to connect it to HIV/AIDS even if it means stepping on some toes. God helps me make connections, too, you know. I think what they want from me is to make sure I can get my group of connections, women and men, through HIV stuff and get them interested in these issues or show up for a protest or something. They know that I know a lot of people, you know, people in agencies and community groups and boards.

Now we turn to Simone. During her first interview, after living with HIV for over two years and embarking on the life reconstruction process, she expressed interest in working with women. Recall from an earlier chapter, she expressed that she was very angry (as many women were) at the circumstances of how she found out she was HIV-positive.

SIMONE: *I would love to be involved with something the women are doing. Mmmm hmmm. Because I have a lot I feel as though I could share with another woman who's been out there, that I've been through the same thing, that's going through the same thing I've been through. And hopefully there's someone that I could share that with out there, to bring in one or two to prevent them from, if they're already where I'm at in life with their health problems. You know, maybe keep them from you know, hurting someone else's life. Or maybe just to save theirs.*

Along with her interest in women and HIV, she also had a strong investment in deterring girls from teen pregnancy. She personally struggled with teen pregnancy in her family, as both of her daughters were pregnant by the age of sixteen. She combined those interests and volunteers at a hospital with a program for high-risk pregnant teens:

I've kind of settled into what I like to do . . . a little one-on-one counseling with the young women. I feel I'm at the hub of what's going on. There is a lot of exciting things progressing. I'm very happy about my activities.

Simone also has helped organize women to attend various women and HIV/AIDS conferences throughout the country. Because she loves kids, she is routinely called to help with childcare either through support groups or from women themselves.

Anna's activities have primarily rested in helping the Latino community in the Detroit metro area. She has been inconsistent in her activities because of her struggles with both drug use and domestic violence. Despite these challenges she has gone through some HIV/AIDS training and has participated in street outreach work with drug users. Her abusive partner's responses to Anna's emerging interests were often not positive or supportive. He did not welcome her interest in promoting safe sex workshops or her interest in getting involved in the newly initiated needle exchange program in Detroit. During her first interview about potential interest in advocacy and other related HIV/AIDS work she said:

ANNA: *Well, I see myself participating in church. Yep. I want to see myself, well now, I'm slowing down. See, I want to do so many things also related to HIV. Like, I want to be a volunteer for HIV. I want to volunteer for HCS [Hispanic Community Support]. But see the guy that I live with, I know that he's not going to let me do that. He's not going to let me be out there passing condoms. That's something that I would love to do, because I think getting AIDS is bad, and there's a lot of shit going on out there. A lot of it too, besides AIDS, there's herpes, gonorrhea, you name it.*

Two years after this initial interview Anna never found her way to church or being active in church. She was, however, one of the main "point people" that Latino organizations called upon in order to talk to small groups about living with HIV/AIDS. Through her own initiative she worked with two owners of local bars on the West Side of Detroit and was able to set up safe sex materials. She still struggles with drug dependency, but has been able to be very productive and active regarding her work around HIV/AIDS issues. She did make significant changes in her personal life; leaving her abusive lover helped her become more involved in other activities. During one of our last interviews, Anna indicated that she preferred a more fluid and flexible approach to working on HIV/AIDS issues:

> The only way I'd do any official advocating is if I was going to work with the youth. I've been asked to do that. I like doing work in other areas though, if truth be told. Even though it is hard for me to go back to certain environments [places where alcohol is served], I feel that is where I am most needed. I know the street and the people who come and go on it. That's where I'm needed.

Activists

> We're fighting for our lives. There's no time to be nice. Even with all the things groups that have accomplished with AIDS—it seems that Detroit is living ten years behind that era. That's why my politics are turning more radical and dramatic.
>
> —Cherise, thirty-two

> I hope when people see my art, they'll realize how comfortable they've become thinking that the U.S. has got AIDS beat. There's nothing further from the truth.
>
> —Shenna, twenty-five

> People respond when you're in your face about what you want and believe . . . like [you were] an irritant. Being an activist is like being a bug that just won't go away.
>
> —Kitt, thirty-three

> Activists help others to see connections whether they want to or not. Most people don't want to see the connections in life.
>
> —Daria, thirty-seven

The women who comprise to this category do so also from self-definition. The "active side" of activism, self-defined by the women, includes engaging in political protests, producing graffiti and counterculture art, and as Shenna said in many interviews, "raising hell."

These women have taken classes in civil disobedience, have interrupted city meetings, and had other encounters that are aimed at getting mainstream society, often defined as "the people in power," to pay attention to their issues. The "people in power" could be thought of as the general public, the state of Michigan, sometimes specifically Detroit African American communities, and non-HIV-positive people—and in Cherise's case, the heterosexual community. The issues that concern activists tend to be an interlocking knot related to broadly defined women's issues, women and HIV/AIDS issues, and HIV/AIDS prevention. One of the things that help to define at least two of the activists is the focus on helping to reshape the image of people with HIV/AIDS. They are more explorative about the political world than both helpers and advocates, and see themselves devoted to the political issues at the edge. Two of the women have some background as advocates.

Cherise first began working as a van driver at Nicole's organization, which allowed her access to the ongoing support group and provided financial support. She was feeling pretty confident about her recent reconciliation with her brother and her family. Cherise was in the process of getting pulled into the advocacy realm through the contacts she was making with Nicole and Nicole's group and the development of her own interests. Moreover, Cherise had been attending an outpatient treatment service and felt her life was stabilizing. She had admitted in previous interviews that being a lesbian at times made her feel very different from the rest of her peers about her HIV status. Cherise was also disgruntled because there were only sporadic services for HIV-positive lesbians, even though there exists an organized black gay and lesbian community.

During the interview about her emerging, interests, she expressed a certain level of boredom working at PPHO.[18] She was in the process of trying new things, like writing an article about being an HIV-positive African American lesbian for a Detroit black gay and lesbian oriented newspaper:

CHERISE: *How is it working here? It's, basically it's just, OK. It's pretty boring to me. Because half the day we're sitting in the office looking at the computer trying to look like we're doing something when we're not. Then there's days like today, which wasn't supposed to be a day like today, that I'm running around everywhere. Sometimes it's fun, I like it. Actually, I like driving, so this is an ideal job for me. I was driving somewhere else, but I was making $4.25 an hour. And I was driving myself to death for eight hours a day. And then, now I'm working here, doing less driving, you know, for you know, more than double what I was getting there. And I'm doing less work, so shit, I love it. I love it. I'm going to go do some training. I'm thinking about going to be a [HIV/AIDS] counselor. There is a counseling and training, HIV-positive and testing training from the second through the sixth. And hopefully, after I'm done with that, I'll be able to get more involved in community aspects of the HIV epidemic. I think there are people out there who need to know that this shit ain't a joke. People like I was. Somebody needs to get to those people, because nobody reached me. You know, and so I think I need to, I want to be the one who reaches out to them, and let them know that this shit ain't no joke.*

A year and a half later after going ahead with the training, then doing some advocacy work (unpaid) at a local substance abuse program that had an HIV/AIDS component, her thoughts had changed about what she wanted for herself, and what she saw as possible:

MICHELE: *So tell me about how being an HIV/AIDS advocate went.*
CHERISE: *It was okay. . . . [nods her head]. Yeah, just okay. I got really restless, no one wanted to do anything which treaded on the toes of someone else. I'm glad I got the experience though. At the same time, or right in there my girlfriend and I started taking this video and film course at a community college and I got all caught up in that. I'm putting together a short video about women with HIV. You know the real deal stuff. We also want to do some stuff on lesbians.*

To go back to your original question, I was interested in getting involved with young people too, and the place I was working at as an advocate/counselor let me plan this event in two high schools which was on safe sex—actually I thought it up, but it involved two other community centers which got more credit than we did—but anything you do with schools will have parents breathing down your neck, there were so many rules and regulations. I can't even tell you. My boss said the program cost too much, and it was too controversial, he cut back the emphasis on kids understanding sexuality—that shit—way back. I said "Controversial? These are the kids we need to learn about this shit." You know, so I had wanted to try to make it an annual program, if I would have stayed there but it just didn't work out. The program was okay. After about eight months of working there I quit so I could pursue these issues from a whole different perspective. Oh, yeah . . . too on my own I hosted a safe sex night for lesbians at Ain't Nobody's Business, which was very successful. We had a great deejay and everything, and I'm more into stuff like that now.

Hey, you never know what's possible until you get your head out of your ass.

Cherise later on went to the National Gay and Lesbian Task Force Conference, where she learned about the philosophy of nonviolent civil disobedience. She continues to be active in the Black gay and lesbian community around HIV issues.

Kitt attributes her interest in activism to her time in treatment and working through an analysis of the reasons why women worked on the street. She said it was then that she began to envision ways to help other young women. Recall from chapter 2 that Kitt was prostituting on the street at a very early age. That was a formative experience for her. While still in outpatient recovery she volunteered at FIT and worked on their Street Outreach Program. She enjoyed interacting with the other staff members, and felt her knowledge about the street was appreciated: "That was the first time someone asked me my opinion about anything related to prostitution." Kitt stated that the FIT group was incredibly supportive of having a former "woman of the streets" on the van shift. They encouraged her to pursue her nursing degree, which she did part-time but stopped. Also, during the time of her FIT volunteer work she read many books on prostitution available in the FIT library. Some of these books had an antiprostitution content. That material heavily influenced Kitt. She credits FIT staff members for introducing her to the writings of black feminists. She acknowledges the time at FIT as her greatest influence for the work she was to do later. "I learned how to think better, read better." She began handling some of the HIV/AIDS administrative component of their Outreach. When not on an FIT shift, Kitt, with the help of a friend, rides around in a car and discusses HIV-risk with women on the street; she calls her work "rough house education." In the long run she would like to develop a program specifically designed to get women out of prostitution. She would like to become involved with antiprostitution organizations. When asked about why she calls herself an activist, she said:

KITT: *You have* [respondent stretched out the word "have"] *to say unpopular things. An activist to me says unpopular things. To be honest I didn't even know what an activist was, let alone people saying that I was one. But activist means to me to be active about something* [moves her hands]. *It's about trying to do something different. Okay, let me start over. Doing the projects I do hasn't hurt anything else in my life, and it hopefully won't in the future. When I'm on the street I know that . . . that's why I think umm I am good at it. I don't like the streets* [determinedly]. *But I know them like that back of my hand, and that's why I can work with those women. I've been on the streets, you know really trying to survive. Other people never felt the cold up close . . . you know they mean well. I've had to live my life on the edge for so long. That's they way it feels like now, it's just home. Street politics, that's what I'm about.*

Kitt disclosed that she often goes through periods of burnout because of her activities. She also has to balance her activities and supporting herself. Women who are activists think about their activities differently from the way the other two groups do, and because they are usually not paid, they have to make specific time for their projects.

One day I met Shenna at a meeting at the Inglewood[19] Public Library—Main Branch office. She was sitting quietly with two other white women and one Latino man. They were in the final stages of discussing a project on HIV/AIDS and literature to coordinate with all the other local branch libraries. Her red hair and freckles seemed understated, and when she spoke she was incredibly polite, directing the conversation to projects that could make a much broader statement about the impact of HIV/AIDS. She suggested the library have particular days devoted to the various groups who were also affected by HIV in the closest city—Detroit. They were less receptive to this idea and seemed visibly uncomfortable as Shenna continued to discuss those groups in detail: drug users, sex workers, gays and lesbians. The person in charge argued that it would be hard to find "literature" written by drug users who had HIV/AIDS. She packed up her things a few minutes early, and when the meeting adjourned, we left, and she said:

> SHENNA: *That was the first project I've been on in a long while which has to do with anything official for this area. Did you see that guy's face when I asked about doing special topics? Those are the people who influence things, so you've got to keep them happy. Actually, they are an okay bunch of people. I've worked with Carlie [one of the women at the meeting] before, on a different project.*

Activism for her, has brought her often "more pain than good." She has been frustrated with political projects both in Detroit and where she grew up, in Inglewood. She struggles to bring her message and her sense of the HIV-positive community to people who would rather not hear it:

> *When you're talking about sheltered white people . . . they're scared. I knew that before I became HIV-positive, but it has been brought home to me when I try to raise issues here. I can hide. Shit I can pack up right now and move into my parents' house and never have to face HIV . . . mostly cause I'm white. But it's affecting us, too. It's not a white black thing, I'm not trying to say that, . . . but rates for white women are going up in the state. I go down to parts of Cass Corridor every once in a while, and there's all these fresh-faced white girls doing heroin. Yeah, and they don't know what the hell they are doing, and chances are quite high they got dirty needles, and they're going to get infected. If not by a needle than from some trick.*
> MICHELE: *So do you do the things you do because you felt that was you on the street? Even though you were not on heroin?*
> SHENNA: *I'm doing certain things because no one cares about those women. White or black. But right now I'm trying to reach those hard-headed mother——, sorry didn't mean to curse. Anyway, I'd like to do something where some of the things I create can make people aware about what risks they face whether they do drugs or not, but especially if they do.*

Through her contacts she created an art fund-raiser where she sponsored herself and three other women to see the traveling AIDS Quilt. Her activism is fueled by anger, and she is currently looking for a way to funnel her energies. She feels that people in the Detroit political scene are humoring women with HIV/AIDS:

> *Yeah, they get you some counseling and then you go and have people mouth off at you at small little conferences. But still, they are not talking about big issues—the Needle Exchange is one exception. That's one good thing Detroit is doing. They need to be talking about women, prevention for kids, people in rural areas [stops abruptly] I know what I need to do—get a Ph.D. like you [laughter from both interviewer and respondent].*

She wants to continue to do creative things that make people aware. Shenna has created many original designs from which she has used to create HIV/AIDS-inspired postcards and posters. Some of the designs on the postcards have captions underneath that say "An HIV+ person is laying on a bed near you." Or, "Stop! Before you do anything else get an HIV test!" She had recently discovered the work of Keith Haring. She tried once to "tag up" graffiti in her neighborhood. She said she went with a friend one night, and only wound up spraying a sign near a store in a strip mall.[20] She spends some of her free time at the Detroit Institute of the Arts (DIA), and thinks she wants to go to college for a degree in the graphic arts: "For the first time I think I could have some sort of focus. Before, I just wanted to go, just to go, because I thought I should."

Shenna's activism is a range of contradictions: "I want to keep focusing on the suburbs where everyone thinks they are safe. But, I also love working with women in Detroit. There the issues are right in your face. Life or death issues. People need it all—affordable housing, safety in their communities, better treatment programs, just about everything." Shenna has made alliances with several other advocates in this study. Often she feels defeated and uncertain of where her activities are going to take her. One project that has been difficult for her to implement is one that would involve a coordination of the malls in the greater Detroit area to provide space or booths for the promotion of materials on HIV/AIDS:

> I basically want them to help on World AIDS Day. Me and some other people are trying to talk with the people who run the malls to get information set up in booths and also to have stores donate materials for a silent auction. Integrate the malls into AIDS service. I don't see why that is such a radical idea but we haven't been able to pull it off yet. Yet, if I wanted to sell funky earrings from some broken down booth—that's not a problem.

She wants to move to New York, Los Angeles, or Atlanta, three places where she feels HIV/AIDS activism is very visible.

Daria was diagnosed in 1991. Around the beginning of 1994, after gaining some ground and some success with recovery for drugs, she slowly moved into advocating for herself. Daria's early sexual trauma was one of the most difficult barriers she had to confront in her process. Because of her own journey, she was able to unravel the complex knot of oppression that she thought accounted for her low self-esteem. She went through HIV/AIDS counseling and training through her program. Daria noted that the beginning of her activism was initiated when she tentatively suggested to a counselor that she wanted to specifically work with HIV-positive women who had been through sexual trauma or assault.

This type of work, though difficult and depressing at times, managed to give Daria a set of new skills. She took other types of life-management classes, and through the help of a caseworker began cofacilitating the program on sexual assault and trauma with a trained therapist. Her interest around sexual survivor issues intensified. Her interests led her to other women in the Detroit HIV-positive community like Julianna and Nicole, who have been very supportive of Daria's efforts. Daria discovered and read many of the classic works on women, sexual abuse, and violence. One of her major contributions to the HIV-positive community was a newsletter about being HIV-positive and being a sexual survivor, which ran for a year. I asked her how she was able to bring that idea to fruition:

> DARIA: *For some time, I just focused on getting basic skills. You can't mouth off about anything if you don't have recovery skills. So I kept getting my act together. And I got this idea to do something for women that hadn't been done before. I suggested a newsletter for women in the HIV community that specifically addressed sexual survivor issues. There are a lot of us out there just weighed down with trying to deal with things that happened to us as little girls. I couldn't believe that no one thought of this before. So I approached six HIV/AIDS groups and said that I was willing to do all the work for it—if they'd give me seed money and small grants so that I could distribute the newsletter. I told them I'd get the contributions, learn layout—I already knew how to use a computer. I promised them the world of what I could do on my own. As it turned out, I needed more help with some things related to the newsletter than I thought—but it was still my baby. I got the contributors—mostly from Detroit and Michigan—and edited some of their stories. It was really a challenge to keep it going.*
>
> MICHELE: *Why do you see yourself as an activist?*
>
> DARIA: *I see connections between what we say we want as a country and what we actually get for our people. In the newsletter, although we focused on where people were, I snuck in facts and statistics about women's vulnerability in this society. I'm not saying that my argument is men against women, but how we all use our power. Little girls aren't empowered in this society to think of their bodies. There's multiple levels that my newsletter tried to get people to think about: silences—their own and others, who we protect in our communities and why.*

She would eventually like to go to school and get a degree in social work.

For the women discussed, activism has been a way for them to bring their own concerns into sharper focus. They do not mind the engagement with the political world. The feeling of being different is what marks Cherise, and to some degree it could be argued that this is true of Shenna because she is a white women with a stigmatized past. Kitt felt different because of her early experiences with prostitution, and Daria is driven by early childhood demons. Activists, perhaps, draw more on their stigmatizing identities than the other two groups. Activists tend to want to be more involved with producing cultural and expressive understandings of HIV/AIDS.

NARRATIVE FEATURES OF PARTICIPATION

This section highlights what types of narrative features emerge from the participation that has been discussed. Given the discussion earlier in the book about intersectional stigma, we might expect that not only the way respondents are active is different from other groups with HIV/AIDS, but also that their participation has a unique set of features. I argue that the features of their activism suggest that they are centered on black females, experiential, and community mandated.

Experiential

The women rely on experientially based knowledge and learning; they take risks and make mistakes. They learn from each other. Most of the women and AIDS activism could fit under the term "experiential," given the recent expansion of large groups of women with HIV/AIDS who are politically active. There have been few established patterns or organizations—women often made it up as they went along (see Dennison 1995; Lockett 1995; Hollibaugh 1995; Carlomusto 1992; Downing 1995; Stoller 1998). For the women of this population, the concept of the experiential also draws from their notions of advocacy and substance abuse treatment.

Many of the women that are active encourage other women and men to be strong, and to give voice to the pain and problems that they encounter. Valerie, who has conducted HIV prevention educational forums in prison, constantly tells women, "How can I stand up and talk about your problem if you won't come and stand beside me and talk about your problems?" Encouraging women (and men) to speak from their own experience and truth is a constant refrain from respondents. This encouragement implies more than speaking from experience; it encourages women to trust themselves and take risks in ways (namely, to take steps on their own behalf) many of them have not done before. Nicole often skillfully draws women out and asks them to translate the skills learned in "the life" into other areas. Of course, she wants to help the woman get off drugs, but she does not invalidate other life experiences. Nicole discussed her philosophy about her skills:

Oh, yeah, because I always say you can turn a negative into a positive. I say the same thing that you did out there [on the street, or in the life], you can do it in recovery, but you just do it in a different way. And I always give this advice, I say, when I was out there I did it all.

People always be talking about me because now it's like I got all these projects that I care about, and all the politics I'm involved. . . . For some of things I get paid, and I get paid from the Engagement Bureau. And I'm well known in the community. And if somebody else wants me to speak, I really don't charge them, but if they want to pay me then I accept it. And so, anyway, people always be talking about how many jobs, and how much I be doing, right? But you know what I tell them? I said, "Well, when I was in my addiction, I had five guys staying in my house selling dope. I'd give this one five dollars and he gave me a rock, I went and sold that for more, and on and on. And so what's the difference?" You know what I'm saying. So I was using that as, well, I did that, I had that many guys in my house rolling [selling crack], well, I might as well do the same thing now and get paid, speak my mind, and have people listen to me. You got

*to use everything you know when you're HIV-positive. You know what I'm saying? So
that's what I do, that's what I tell some of the women.*

Her unorthodox philosophy is something that resonates with many of the
women who have come from drug-using backgrounds. Respondents are
also able to get women to identify with the more active aspects of being "in
the life." Respondents discourage passivity among the women. Because of
the "anything goes that works" approach, women are encouraged by each
other to discover a range of talents and revalue some of their survival skills.
Moreover, because women move back and forth among their roles, there is
a greater flexibility and transferring of skills from one area to the other.

Black Female Centered

The idea that the political work respondents engage in is black female-
centered comes from three observations: (1) the women recognize the
larger inequities African American women face in Detroit and Michigan
in the struggle around HIV/AIDS; (2) the people many respondents come
into contact with (grass-roots leadership within HIV/AIDS circles and in
other positions) are often African American women; and (3) respondents
are continually in an environment that keeps them aware that the usefulness of the programs they develop has to in some way relate to the large
African American population who is HIV-positive. Moreover, many of
the respondents have also been influenced by basic concepts espoused in
multiracial feminist or womanist thought.[21] These concepts often involve
ideas about the sharing of power and empowerment issues for women of
color. The respondents are also aware of the local and national context of
how HIV/AIDS affects the African American community.

We know HIV/AIDS organizing has made people brutally aware of
seemingly intractable class and race differences. These differences have at
times overwhelmed activists and advocates alike (see Schneider and Stoller
1995; Stoller 1998). There are definitely tensions of these kinds for the
women in Detroit as they struggle over access to groups, monies, and activities. Despite this however, the base of leadership remains black female
led and centered, which is unusual for a group of stigmatized women.

GEORGIA: *I know that it's a bit of cliché to say that black women bear the brunt of
everything but we do. When I was first starting out it was only black women I knew and
saw who were dealing with this. Now we got white sisters, Latina sisters—[as an aside]—
I'm still trying to work on my Spanish. But the black women are hard hit by this disease.*

The caseloads for Julianna, Nicole, and Charlene include women of various ethnicities, but overwhelmingly they are African American. Many of
the primary contacts they have with other social workers, other activists,

advocates, or helpers are African American. Often a woman coming into contact with services will meet African American women in almost every stage of this process: substance abuse counselor, peer advocate, HIV/AIDS counselor, support staff, other women in support groups. For some of the women, it might be the first time they have experienced other black women in supervisory and peer group leader roles.

Nicole's concern for women also comes from seeing the promise of services for women with HIV which do not pan out year after year:

I would like to see more women's services come about. Every time they start a women service, somebody's doing something with the money. I'm serious, I know this for a fact. And they start something for women, and then they don't finish it. They don't follow through on women like they do for the men. I would love to see more services so women can take their children. The children have to learn to grow up in the process, too. See right now, a lot of the children are coming from dysfunctional families. So it's like, even though the mother is getting educated, the children need to be reeducated, the mother needs to be reeducated. There needs to be more trade programs where women can just take their children and go. They can be in day care there and the mother can be there. Transportation is another issue. And so it's hard for ladies right now. Especially a mother with children. A mother with children wants to do these things. Like for women who are HIV-positive, they just want a women's HIV-positive group. They don't want to have to share the group. They need to speak on different issues. They need to speak on the issues about the man that gave them HIV, and they've been sitting at home all these years just with that one man. It's different for women than it is for men. They just think that it's just a gay thing. Black heterosexual men don't want to stand up. They don't. They feel ashamed. So if the man's ashamed, how do you expect the wife's going to feel or the woman's going to feel if the man can't stand up? I've been seeing relationships here lately where the man is still in denial. The woman can accept it, but the man is in denial. And he gave it to the woman.

Nicole often stresses a color-blind approach, but has a hard time maintaining that approach when there are scarce resources and other groups, including those of predominantly white gay men, who are reluctant to work with groups that face discrimination. During the time of this research in Detroit there were some key committees that had a disproportionate number of gay white men who made decisions without, in the opinions of Nicole and others, taking into account that the demographics of the disease suggested channeling more resources to helping underserved populations: minority women and others including inmates, minority men who sleep with men but do not identify as gay or bisexual, and drug users:

No, see one of the things that I'm glad about my mother, she never brought us up with stereotypes about nobody is better than us, we're all the same. She said, white people didn't do nothing to us because it's what you do to yourself and what you do for yourself.

I've raised my son the same way. White people ain't doing nothing to you. If you want to get it, you go out there and get it. You are just as good as anybody else. I don't see AIDS as being a color thing, but I do see it looking like this—when I sit at the table, HIV and AIDS are hitting the Afro-American community more, but it's more white gay men sitting at the table. Yeah. That's where I see the color line at. And the bottom line at that for black women . . . until we as blacks start standing up more, we won't be recognized.

Almost the entire first wave of active HIV-positive women in Detroit was African American. This means that black women often set the level of discussion and the cultural setting. Although the respondents often evoke "women of color" as a category, many concrete examples are used in reference to African American women. Respondents are very aware of the high rates of HIV/AIDS in the black community and there is networking within the black communities (when and where possible) around HIV/AIDS issues. Other women, including Anna and Shenna, have not felt threatened by this black-female-centered feature of HIV/AIDS work. Anna had this to say when asked about black women and HIV/AIDS issues:

No, I like it. At first it took me awhile to get used to . . . that's one of things I've had to accept with this HIV, it . . . um you have to be open to people, new people . . . ideas. I like being among Mexicans, no doubt, but I've learned a lot through many of the black women.

Community Mandate

Through their participation within a broadly defined HIV/AIDS community, they begin to receive what could be called a community mandate. They are rewarded for their service and effort locally and at the state level. For their hard work, and commitment, local elites, community actors, reporters, and policy makers, among others, often recognize the women. Whether it is awards from agencies, the city, representatives, or council members, over time many respondents are noticed. The outcome of this recognition can be broadly understood as a community mandate (Gilkes 1980, 1988, 1994). This makes them feel proud, as they have tangible evidence of their work, and it keeps them committed to their often unnoticed difficult struggles. Over time, I argue that this sense of a community mandate helps to reduce the type of stigmatized treatment that some respondents receive. With recognition comes increased visibility and contact, factors that help to change people's perceptions and responses to stigmatized women with HIV/AIDS.

There is a sense of shared activity and purpose among the respondents. Several women have developed broad social networks, have traveled, and are well known by other women in Detroit and throughout the Midwest. About organizing other women across the country one respondent stated,

"We have to be here for each other. We can do it for each other if we can stop being shamed not to talk. We need each other."

This sense of connection that allows for personal and political transformation recalls Ackelsberg's (1988) assertion that scholars rethink traditional models of gender participation. She refutes the traditional models of participation composed of atomistic individuals who are unconnected to others. She reformulates the model to instead view women as political actors through their connections that then bring them into broader political activity (Ackelsberg 1988; Naples 1998).

For subordinate groups there is another realm that women and other groups interact in, often described as the private, the familiar, or the intimate. This is a space that has tended to be devalued when thinking about politics. McCourt (1977), in her discussion of white working-class women who became politically active in their communities against toxic waste, discusses the processes by which the women came to regard each other. She suggests that "community" is often a catchall phrase that denotes commonality, consensus decision making, and agreement. She concludes, however that this word does not entirely capture the transformation of her group of women's struggles and significant regard for the other. She posits that with her group "communion" exists, as opposed to the static concept of community.

She suggests that the idea of communion captures the concept that alternatives do happen when women work together on issues of importance. Unfortunately, this intriguing concept is briefly mentioned and then not elaborated upon by McCourt. Because of the life-and-death types of issues that these respondents face on a day-to-day level, there is the possibility that their working together in some way creates a kind of communion that allows for not only politics, but other ways of being and experiencing each other in the world than was currently possible prior to their coming together.

It precisely in the ways the women extend themselves through their roles as workers, activists, advocates and helpers that create overlapping spheres of authority and networks that enlarge opportunities and possibilities. The ability to sustain ties with groups they are interested in while surviving a life-threatening disease allows for lasting connections to be made.

## CHAPTER EIGHT

Looking to the Future: Struggle and Commitment for Stigmatized Women with HIV/AIDS

> *Telling collective stories is one way in which we as social scientists can use our skills and privileges to give voice to those whose narratives have been excluded from public domain and civic discourse.*
> —Laurel Richardson, *Writing Strategies*

COLLECTIVE STORIES

THE WOMEN whose stories are told in this book—HIV-positive women from stigmatized pasts who became politically active—represent a new thread of participation in contemporary political life. Individually, their early histories were daunting. Additionally, the hegemonic influences of race, class, and gender predominate in describing their life challenges. But the ability to change the seemingly irreversible avalanche of negative life circumstances dominates the majority of the book. Their collective story narrates a complex series of events stemming from both the public and private sphere that has helped them transform themselves and the lives of many other HIV-positive people in Detroit and the surrounding Metro area. Richardson (1990) suggests that the power of telling collective stories lies in its potential to shape collective identity (for those listening to the stories), and in a most optimistic manner creates the promise for collective solutions to social problems. Collective solutions to the dilemmas of women and HIV/AIDS will require attention, commitment, and social change.

This book takes issue with the traditional framing of politics and the invisibility of marginalized/stigmatized women's political awakening. First, to understand stigmatized women's political involvement, we must broaden our notion of what is political and examine the circumstances that lead women to act on behalf of themselves and their communities. Scholars can only *gain* by such an expansion in the definition of politics. Scholars gain from this expanded definition by being able to observe and record the multifaceted responses to injustices that galvanize women (see Ackelsberg 1988; Bookman and Morgen 1988; Naples 1998).

The evolution in political consciousness that a respondent experiences is a change first experienced by the self, which then moves out through her community. Ackelsberg suggests that active participation and resistance "often [engender] a broader consciousness of both the nature and dimensions of social inequality, and the power of people united to confront and change it" (1988, 307). Respondents were able to identify that they were marginalized and stigmatized through acquiring the HIV/AIDS virus, act on that identification, and communicate that knowledge to others. Marginalized and stigmatized women need a place from which to speak about contradiction, resistance, and agency. These women challenge timely ideas about former female lawbreakers but they also challenge notions about the route to political socialization and about what is possible for people labeled deviant.

Second, I began the book with the argument that it is necessary to understand these women's lives, before and during the HIV/AIDS crisis, through the framework of intersectional stigma. Intersectional stigma presents an innovative theoretical apparatus in conceptualizing the complexity of respondents' politicization process. Stigma, I have argued, as it intersects with social location provides researchers with useful ways to study manifestations of inequality as well as barriers to participation. Stigma suggests people can occupy the margins of society with qualitatively different types of experiences. Stigma condemns and confers power. HIV stigma is a totalizing type of stigma, developed in local and global contexts; it is predicated on issues of difference, sexuality, and taboo. HIV-stigma developed along axes of inequality in U.S. society.

What this research demonstrates is that HIV stigma and social status converged to shape women's experiences with HIV and, later, participation in dramatically different ways than have been previously observed. Intersectional stigma impacts resources including time, money, and civic skills. This concept is particularly useful in moving beyond the mantra of race, class, and gender, which at times suggests a "sameness" of experience for all working-class Latina women (for example), and pushes us as social scientists to engage with other complex ways in which societal rewards and punishments are allocated. As stated before, respondents share some similarities to other groups of HIV-positive people, but their political evolution was distinct because of intersectional stigma.

Third, life reconstruction was a specific, ongoing process for the respondents. The two components of life reconstruction are recovery and gender identity/consciousness. The life reconstruction process helped women redefine themselves. While women were highly disadvantaged when it came to accessing traditional political resources, the life reconstruction process allowed them to develop and seek out both external and internal resources.

Recovery afforded the women an opportunity to deal with their addiction, and during the (recovery) process they often discovered and developed some nontraditional resources, like spirituality. Recovery introduced them to the language of self-advocacy, which they would later draw on in their political activities. The language of advocacy reaffirmed to them the importance of taking control of one's life and demanding dignity as human beings.

After becoming HIV-positive, the women reconstructed aspects of their gender identity. This reconstruction included valuing themselves outside other primary roles as mother, partner, and worker as well as moving away from an exclusive focus on racial identification. They also had to deal with sexuality in new and multiple ways including, taking responsibility for their sexuality and becoming sexually self-educated. This process also included valuing and spending time with other women. Respondents, in dealing with their HIV-positive status, had to be willing to explore the sexual "landscapes" in which they had been stigmatized, including childhood sexual trauma and past issues of sex work. Additionally, I argue that dealing with sexual abuse and trauma began to provide a language and vocabulary by which women could begin to understand the concept of women as a social category, and also helped them to see that other women, very much like them (women of color, drug users, relatively poor) also experienced similar phenomena.

This gender aspect of life reconstruction was vital for future political development. This second phase of life reconstruction played a significant role in contributing to the development of a "public voice." Moreover, I demonstrated that women like Billy Jean, who did not fully undertake the life reconstruction process, faced numerous obstructions in continuing her advocacy work.

This research has also highlighted an area that social scientists have traditionally overlooked in understanding barriers to women's political participation. The important role of sexual abuse and dealing with sexual abuse by respondents was examined in chapter 5. Dealing with their sexual abuse and the stigma attached to it played a crucial role in helping these women become confident people, people better able to navigate in the social world. Understanding the importance of sexual abuse and sexual trauma has been introduced into public discourse only in the last fifteen years. Much of this research has been conducted in the areas of psychology and feminist theory (see Barry 1995; Hoigard and Finstad 1992 for prostitution; Boyd et al. 1994, 1993a, 1993b; Maher and Curtis 1992; Purnell 1996 for women drug users). However, the majority of social scientists have been slow to develop conceptualizations about sexual trauma and its possible interference in many types of public activities—including politics.

The mapping of advocate, activist, and helper were helpful markers in assessing the roles women played in their communities. The idea of blended and overlapping roles has been a way to get at the distinct phenomenon of paid employment, volunteer work, and community activism. Blended and overlapping roles also allow a window into the ways women have adapted traditional roles to suit their specific needs and desires. Although fraught with tension, these roles continue to be a source of strength and pride for many of the women. The diversity of these roles should suggest that low-income/marginalized women's activism is a prism worth further exploration. This in-depth focus revealed how their political transformations were community focused, black female led, and personally experiential.

Fourth, I have highlighted the challenges of representing stigmatized women's participation. Throughout the book there was recognition that as a researcher I was simultaneously trying to understand the experiences of the HIV-positive women *and* use their experiences to broaden the definition of what constitutes politics, specifically informal political participation. There were moments of disjuncture between how the women understood their political and social world, their activities within it, and how I understood those same activities. In particular, this tension was most apparent in trying to account for the activities of the helpers and some of the advocate-oriented women. I did listen to the ways in which several of the women refused to view their activities within a political sphere. As a researcher, however, I was also motivated to contextualize and position their struggles within a larger historical and social perspective informed by various academic, feminist, and medical discourses. This repositioning of their narratives created a broader analysis, one that is recognizable by others besides the respondents. Borland discusses the challenges of creating what she calls "second-level" narrative from data:

> To refrain from interpretation by letting the subjects speak for themselves seems to me an unsatisfactory if not illusory solution. For the very fact that we constitute the initial audience for the narratives we collect influences the way in which our collaborators will construct their stories (1991, 64).

What is most useful about this tension between myself and the respondents is that it dramatizes the ways in which people can inhabit the world, affect change, and create meaning for themselves without necessarily using or drawing on dominant or accepted ideas about those activities. As a researcher, I have made my job the analysis to think through these tensions and represent them as clearly to the reader as I can. Presenting the array of women's experiences speaks to the challenges in satisfactorily and inclusively defining participation. Moreover, the research also points to the need for complex understandings of the "why" and the "how" of participation, and the forms that participation takes as it intersects the public sphere.

Policy, Prevention, and Treatment Implications

This book raises two main questions: How can society create a different future for stigmatized HIV-positive women? What are the policy implications of this research?

Women with HIV/AIDS continue to challenge the contemporary American understanding of issues related to stigmatization and marginality. HIV/AIDS and its effect on women reflect other long-standing cracks in our political and social system. Although targeted punitive measures aimed at women with HIV/AIDS have slightly abated, the interrelationships of drugs, race, and stigma continue to govern the popular imagination about HIV/AIDS and women in this country. Indeed, recent surveys of American attitudes toward PWAs (people with AIDS) suggest that although overt expressions of stigmatization has declined, "one fifth of those surveyed still feared PWAs and one sixth expressed disgust or supported public naming of PWAs" (Herak, Capitanio, Widaman, 2002, 375). Moreover, Herak and his colleagues found that not only have more subtle and less overt forms of stigma lingered, but that many people are apt to blame people who contract HIV through either drug use or sex (Herak, Capitanio, Widaman 2002).

Changing the discourse around sex, race, drugs, HIV/AIDS, and stigma is a formidable challenge for us all. National dialogues about stigma in relation to HIV/AIDS should be a priority. Furthermore, public health efforts targeted at destigmatizing people with HIV/AIDS would also contribute to creating tolerance. Valdiserri offers a sobering wake-up call for the public health profession in acknowledging the impact of HIV/AIDS stigma:

> Stigma is a complicated issue that has deep roots in the convoluted domains of gender, race, ethnicity, class, sexuality, and culture. Granted, it is not easily understood, nor is it readily addressed. But public health practitioners must not shy away from the subject of stigma, thinking it is outside the scope of public health or beyond the reach of their capabilities. . . . To ensure these essential services in the context of HIV prevention and care, there is no question that we must all—every single segment of the public health community—confront the impact of HIV/AIDS stigma (2002, 342).

This research has implications for policy makers and the public health community concerned with developing fair policies regarding HIV/AIDS. To address multiply stigmatized female populations affected by HIV/AIDS, policy makers must pay attention to the ways in which different groups of women are socially located. Differently socially located groups of women will benefit from policies that will help them access local resources, including health care and substance abuse treatment. Furthermore, local city and state programs that provide programming for the empowerment of HIV-positive women should continue to be developed and funded. This includes workshops and conferences, classes, and the promotion of "paid activism."

Additionally, early identification of socially vulnerable women with HIV/AIDS is crucial. Linking them to programs (substance abuse treatment and others,—e.g., community programs) that incorporate a therapeutic approach that focuses attention to helping the whole person (not just on one facet of a problem) will also help facilitate interest in informal political participation around HIV/AIDS. Women in these situations are looking for ways to make their lives stable and functional, and well-designed programs have the capacity to help them acquire stability. Programs that help women make conceptual links across race, class, and gender and that emphasize the role of their social location in relation to the HIV/AIDS virus are also vitally needed.

This work suggests further research on HIV-positive women struggling with substance abuse issues. Women with the HIV/AIDS virus who are current or former substance abusers constitute a particularly vulnerable population.

Treatment programs and specialized programs that support women with HIV that I have examined during the course of my research typically shy away from discussions of the macrostructural factors that contribute to drug use and/or the transmission of HIV/AIDS. Given my findings and extended work with stigmatized HIV-positive women, I would encourage a rethinking of these traditional, depoliticized approaches. Stigmatized HIV-positive women often face a hostile political discourse. Thus, helping stigmatized HIV-positive women make sense of that discourse is desirable and would enable them to better confront (and name) the forces that seek to impede their progress. Even more effort is needed to help this population of women with the HIV/AIDS virus cope with the multiple strains they face, including recovery from drug use, (usually) limited economic resources, and the damaging isolating effects of stigma.

Of course we wish to reduce the experience of stigma and marginality for women with HIV/AIDS and increase useful resources. But for intersectionally stigmatized women, it is not only getting them into treatment and medical care that is important, but also helping them to redirect stigma and participate in programs for their overall empowerment. For women with a history of sex work, troubled relationships, and primarily negative experiences with other women, it may be harder to trust and support women. From a treatment and intervention standpoint, this research indicates that any encouragement to help HIV-positive women take responsibility for their sexual health and sexual empowerment and support the process of life reconstruction could have positive long-term effects. Therefore, the continued development of treatment programs with pro-woman or woman friendly aspects embedded into an overall program would be useful for HIV-positive women.

It also strongly suggests that medical providers and human service workers receive further training in dealing with vulnerable and stigmatized HIV-positive populations.

Effective social change relies on both traditional and nontraditional forms of political activity. As chapter 7 demonstrated, many women understand the traditional political sphere as often existing outside of the world they live in. This can have a negative impact for furthering social change for the issues they are most concerned about. It also presents troubling questions about the way people understand their ability to influence political systems.

While there is no way to eliminate stigma, many women with HIV across the United States have found ways to become *visible* as people with HIV to their families, their communities, and sometimes to politicians. Because what we know about women with HIV/AIDS and political organizing/empowerment is still in a formative state it is difficult to draw hard-and-fast conclusions about the future (see Schneider and Stoller 1995; Stoller 1998). There is evidence to suggest that North American women who face multiple stigmas and are HIV-positive *are* beginning to mobilize on their own behalf (Stoller 1998). These groups would include women who are intravenous drug users, prisoners, and homeless women who are HIV-positive (see Friedman and Alicea 2001; Stoller 1998). Understanding HIV-positive women's struggles to redefine themselves and their communities will be a key feature in understanding how marginalized populations participate in confronting the HIV/AIDS epidemic in the coming years.

The experiences of women with HIV/AIDS who use or have used drugs are still part of an ongoing investigation. I have tried to put forth that to understand various forms of political participation, we as researchers have to be "willing to step into the complicated maze of experience that renders 'ordinary' folks so extraordinarily multifaceted, diverse, and complicated" (Kelley 1994, 4). The HIV/AIDS virus provides the opportunity for us to rethink what we understand about how women change their lives and how seemingly impossible odds act as a catalyst for that change.

Appendix

This appendix describes the various programs, groups, agencies, and institutions mentioned throughout the book.

Brightline Hospital

A major hospital on the west side of Detroit. The hospital has a special clinic named Care for You. The clinic specializes in services for women with high-risk pregnancies, which can include conditions ranging from a woman's age and issues of infertility to substance abuse problems.

Females in Trouble (FIT)

A nonprofit organization sponsors programs geared toward the self-empowerment of girls and women of the greater Detroit area. The services include a teenage homeless shelter, a mentoring program, and a street outreach program.

Hispanic Community Support (HCS)

A nonprofit organization that provides a diversity of services to the Latino communities of the greater Detroit area.

Hope For Us

A city-sponsored program that serves HIV-positive people. The program provides testing for the HIV/AIDS virus, counseling, and outpatient services for HIV-positive people.

Life Help

A publicly funded substance abuse treatment service center. The center provides outpatient treatment services for alcohol and drug use as well as various types of therapeutic counseling.

New Day For Us

A small in-patient residential treatment program that supports women with HIV/AIDS who are struggling to meet the demands of everyday living.

Parker Hospital

A midsized hospital located on the east side of Detroit.

Partnership and Participation in Health Organization (PPHO)

A nonprofit organization that runs several types of services for HIV-positive people throughout the Detroit metro area. The services are two-tiered. They assist

HIV-positive clients in accessing medical treatment and social services. The other tier works on behalf of HIV-positive people as a liaison between other community groups involved in HIV/AIDS issues and city agencies. Although they serve both men and women, the women's services are the most comprehensive program of its kind in the Detroit metro area.

Sharon's Place

A substance abuse treatment center that serves women on the west side of Detroit.

The Engagement Bureau

A program sponsored by the city that coordinates HIV/AIDS education and outreach throughout the Detroit Metro area. They maintain a list of men and women who are willing to speak about their experiences living with HIV/AIDS. They provide speakers for many different types of institutions, including schools, prisons, and community centers.

Notes

CHAPTER ONE: THE POLITICS OF INTERSECTIONAL STIGMA
FOR WOMEN WITH HIV/AIDS

1. All the names of the respondents, their friends, other informants, and names of agencies, and institutions (except the Herman Keifer Detroit Department of Health) mentioned are pseudonyms. See the appendix for a description of the various agencies, community groups, programs, and institutions referred to throughout the book.

2. My use of the term *sex work* is grounded in the presuppositions and arguments scholars and activists have advanced in the last two decades. One of the most important arguments put forth is that sex work chiefly constitutes an economic activity. Activities that encompass the domain of sex work include, but are not limited to: erotic dancing, phone sex, escort services, fetish work, massage, pornography, and street-level sex (or what most people would call prostitution). Sexual activities are varied in all of these arenas. Sex workers can be men, women, or transgendered people. The term *sex work* can allude to power, performance, and other aspects of sexuality (see Chapkis 1997; Jenness 1993; McClintock 1993; Nagle 1997; Queen 1997). Carol Leigh, a.k.a. Scarlot Harlot, argues she first coined the term sex work:

> I INVENTED SEX WORK. Not the activity, of course. The term. This invention was motivated by my desire to reconcile my feminist goals with the reality of my life and the lives of the women I knew. I wanted to create an atmosphere of tolerance within and outside the women's movement for women working in the sex industry. (Leigh 1997, 225)

Though respondents did not use this term to refer to their activities, the term encompasses the range of activities engaged in throughout their lives. Using this term is an attempt to situate a much broader understanding about women who smoke crack cocaine and engage in sexual service activities. Respondents described a wide range of feelings toward their practice of sex work.

3. The term HIV stands for Human Immunodeficiency Virus (HIV). AIDS stands for the Acquired Immunodeficiency Syndrome (AIDS). The HIV/AIDS virus suppresses the body's immune system. Alonzo and Reynolds (1995) provide a precise and concise summary of the HIV/AIDS virus and its physical manifestations.

4. The term "female lawbreaker" is a sociologically derived term used to denote the range of women's criminalized activities and behavior (see Maher 1992). Using this term acknowledges that many of the activities the respondents have engaged in are illicit and illegal. The term has also been used by feminist researchers as a way of complicating the context of women's agency in social relations analyzed in local terrains. A new line of research is concerned with interrogating how various practices become coded as deviant and criminalized and how the process of criminalization relates to race, class, and gender inequities (see Davis 2003; Tonry and Petersilia 2000).

5. The term *political* is used throughout the book to define activities that include both conventional and unconventional aspects of what is commonly referred to as political participation. In the second section of this chapter there is a lengthy

discussion of the types of activities the women are involved in, and how many of the activities (e.g., community work) intersect with both the private and public spheres.

6. "Women of color" is often a conflictual and problematic term. It has been used to connote a category of women that have been the recipients of racial and ethnic discrimination. It has also been used to connote the *affinity* of groups of women with certain cultural experiences under complex systems of oppression. Its usage has referred to African Americans, Asian Americans, Caribbean Americans, Native Americans, Chicanas, Latinas, and Pacific Islanders. This term, however, is not limited to these groups. Depending on the context, it has been used to suggest *similarity* of experience among Jewish, Maori, and Aboriginal women. I am using it here in its more general academic usage (which could be thought of as "women of color of the United States"). Throughout the rest of the analysis, I will refer to the ethnicity of a woman where appropriate.

7. I am thinking of the types of narratives about lower-income women that emerged in public discourse throughout the late eighties and nineties, including the public hysteria over the welfare "queen," immigration, and drug use in inner cities and the moral outrage over women producing "crack babies." Reeves and Campbell (1994) provide a compelling discussion about how various news shows during the late 1980s and early 1990s depicted "crack babies." These depictions, they argue, contributed less to understanding what types of medical problems might exist for infants born addicted to crack cocaine, but more about the ideological portrayal of female drug users as "unfit mothers" contributing to the deterioration of society. Campbell (2000) provides an excellent overview of contemporary drug policy narratives and their impact on lower-income women and especially women of color.

These narratives have contributed to punitive policies regarding the distribution of various types of state benefits including Medicare and welfare (in relation to restricting childbirth as well as drug use) (see Zachary-Jordan 2001). The targeting and imprisoning of pregnant female drug users, and requests for mandatory HIV/AIDS testing of pregnant women have appeared in legislative debates in many states (Zerai and Banks 2002; Campbell 2000; Maher 1992; Paltrow 1990).

8. In the United States, it is estimated that close to one million people are infected with the virus. Dr. Phillip Rosenberg, citing the trends of the early nineties, had this to say about the spread of the disease:

> As of January 1993, prevalence was highest among young adults in their late twenties and thirties and among minorities. An estimated 3 percent of black men and 1 percent of black women in their thirties were living with HIV-infection as of that date. If infection rates remain at these levels, HIV must be considered *endemic* in the United States. (1995, 1373, emphasis added)

9. Gilkes (1980) draws on sociological insights into the community worker as an occupational role.

10. Naples's work (1999) discusses how for women in her study, mothering encompasses more than "nurturing work" of kin and includes social activism. Mothering practices shape their definitions of community work.

11. Later in the chapter, I fully discuss the women and HIV/AIDS literature. I will, however, raise one point now. Schneider and Stoller (1995) pay particular attention to explicating the ways in which women's skills and activities within HIV/AIDS leadership are made visible. While they are able to generally identify some

gendered areas, they do not present reasons about what might make these activities unique, or not unique, in a political context. It is clear that globally, HIV-positive women have responded in a variety of ways to the societal challenges of being infected, including building and using new skills. However, scholars have not satisfactorily explored how HIV-positive women understand, construct, or use political power. The focus on roles in this research delves into those experiences, providing a more complete picture of how some women navigate the political sphere.

Understanding the reasons why women with HIV/AIDS do or do not identify with politics also provides some explanatory power toward ideas about how people perceive the larger political system. Role structure and its intersection with community work has been an unexamined aspect of HIV-positive women's participation.

12. In the twentieth century with the advent of various social movements, there has been a tendency, particularly in the United States, to politicize one's identity. The concept of "identity politics," or the embracing of one aspect (or multiple aspects) of one's identity in order to build community and politically participate, has been central in marginalized people's struggles for equal rights and other political freedoms. I would argue that identity politics does not constitute the definitive, central manifestation of the women's community work.

People with HIV/AIDS have struggled to become visible in a self-defined way. They have had to embrace the term HIV-positive person, which has brought solace, political visibility, and solidarity. The women in this group do not, however, conceptualize their political activity solely through an "HIV identity" lens. This is an analytical distinction worth following, because it goes against the grain of the current conceptualization of identity and political activity.

13. The phrase "face-to-face work" is derived from sociological notions about the human importance placed on social relations, which result from interactive work between the self and others (see Goffman 1959).

14. For the sake of clarity, I am focusing here on North American HIV-positive women's activism. Schneider and Stoller (1995) explore activism globally. Within research, policy, and practice there has been a split between focusing on issues internationally or within the United States (see Long and Ankrah 1996; Sherr, Hawkins, and Bennett 1996).

15. Amber Hollibaugh (1995) provides an excellent discussion of how lesbians have dealt with being seen as a "no risk group." Stoller (1998) provides a typology detailing four ways lesbians have responded to the HIV/AIDS virus.

16. This distinction is not to draw hard-and-fast rules between academics and activists; rather, it is to suggest that activists usually have different goals in explicating the social and political role of women with HIV/AIDS than do academics.

17. This concept has been developed within black and Chicana feminist thought (see Moraga and Anzandula 1981). Frances Beale, an African American woman, was one of the first in the modern women's movement to critique the Black Power movement, citing the "double jeopardy" of one's race and gender (Daly and Stephens 1994). This analysis was furthered by the Combahee River Collective (1979). The two main points that developed early on were that specific attention to the relations of race, class, and gender were important, and that if attention was not given to them, then an understanding of unequal power relations could not be advanced (Daly and Stephens 1994).

18. Crenshaw (1989) first coined the term "intersectionality."

19. Although Crenshaw (1997) is specifically developing these paradigms to understand and study women of color's intersectional experiences of violence, I would argue the paradigms are quite useful in other substantive contexts.

20. An example Crenshaw (1997) provides that underscores the complexity and constraints of intersectionality is that of battered women. All battered women want to escape from violent conditions. From casual observation one might view battering as primarily about complex relations of unequal power between men and women (or same-sex couples). She suggests differences between heterosexual battered white women and heterosexual battered women of color. She argues that although heterosexual battered women of color suffer under gender subordination (from the battering of a male partner), because of illiteracy, poverty, lack of job skills (structural inequalities that women of color are *more likely* to face than white women), this phenomenon takes on a different experience. The category of "battered woman" intersects within class and race hierarchies in individual women's lives; the racial subordination (or social pressure) women face may suggest to them that they cannot leave their partner because (1) they may believe police and law enforcement systems unfairly discriminate against men of color or (2) they may be immigrant women who are unable to access services. These and other factors might make it difficult for a woman of color to leave an abusive relationship, and also pose challenges to a community to develop specific intervention programs. This viewpoint of intersectionality has specific consequences in developing prevention and treatment strategies for domestic violence programs. Richie (1996) provides an incredibly insightful argument of how the early "violence against women" movement splintered communities of color. This stems from the fact that organizers and proponents did not focus on the complexity of race and class dynamics, and instead chose to focus on one group of women's experiences.

21. I have found Charlton's (1998) discussion on the inability of stigma to properly theorize about disability oppression because of a lack of attention to difference useful. He argues that attention must be given to understanding specific ways in which stigma crosscuts other identities and is linked with other material resources.

22. "Sex-for-crack exchange" is a popular term among criminologists and researchers of substance use (see Inciardi, Lockwood, and Potteigier 1993). Sex-for-crack exchange refers to a bartering system of sexual services for crack cocaine. This focus on sex-for-crack exchange often obscures women's prostitution/sex work histories before drug use, the historical fact that there has always been an element of sex for drug exchange, and an analysis of women's beliefs and motivations about engaging in any kind of sexual service for money or drugs or both (Berger 1998; Bourgois and Dunlap 1993; Maher 1997).

23. Scholars have noted that with the almost complete collapse of the urban prostitution markets due to crack cocaine, the old stereotypical self-indulgent and flamboyant pimp has been replaced with a drug-using man who is out for sole personal gain and has little interest in providing stability for a woman or her children. Researchers have noted that there were often unspoken rules about what a pimp would do for one of the women in his "stable," including providing food, clothing, housing, and sometimes being involved in the raising of children. In the new crack economy with cutthroat prices, rapid addiction, and high profits, men taking over the role of the pimp had no interest in these older terms of agreement. Consequently, a street

prostitute quickly reached almost unheard of degrees of impoverishment (Inciardi 1993; Ratner 1993).

24. See Ratner (1993) for a full account of the names of the different types of places where buying drugs was also intertwined with prostitution.

25. These issues are discussed through the concept of a HIV/AIDS stigma trajectory (see Alonzo and Reynolds 1995).

26. As Patton (1994) notes, HIV/AIDS was first characterized by the media and certain health officials as a disease of "deviants," thus lulling the general public into believing that only certain types of sexual encounters were risky and only certain groups were at risk for contracting the HIV/AIDS virus. We now know that everyone is at *physiological* risk for contracting the HIV/AIDS virus.

27. Allen Brandt (1985) develops this argument.

28. I am indebted to Kim Lane Scheppele and Martha Feldman for their insights on this point.

29. Some gay men have written about multiple levels of stigma. Many of these critiques have come from gay men of color who deal with race and class issues in relation to the predominately white gay male community (for gay men of color critiques see Hemphill 1991).

30. Perrow and Gullien (1990) discuss the founding of the Gay Men's Health Crisis. Cohen (1993) provides a lively and critical discussion of gay male resource utilization versus that of other outsider groups during the first wave of HIV/AIDS.

31. Some research has suggested that women of color are often engaged in the most brutal form of sex work—street-level sex work (Arnold 1990; Delacoste and Alexander 1987). The brutality lies in the fact that street-level sex work is a less protected, less insulated, and a more stigmatized form of sex work, especially when drugs are implicated.

32. WHISPER and other organizations that oppose prostitution ran, and still run, newsletters that discuss women of color in the sex work industry.

33. One of the major exceptions to this is the history of the activist Gloria Lockett. Lockett is an African American woman who along with primarily other African American women founded California Prostitutes' Education Project (Cal-PEP). This was a highly successful organization. She then went on to help change the mission of the organization by turning to HIV/AIDS awareness and educational work. For a thorough history about Lockett see Stoller 1998 and an interview in Chapkis 1997.

34. It could be argued that because black women's sexual identity, in particular, has historically been constructed as easy, worthless, nonrapeable, and nonhuman (see Collins 1990; Davis 1981, 1989), claiming a public sexual identity, or "whoredom," would be very difficult. It is hard for a black woman to claim the public space as a whore, sex worker, or other rebellious sexual identity—primarily because this has been a central depiction in public and popular culture (see Crenshaw 1997; hooks 1994; Wallace 1990, 1992). This difficulty could be described as the historical ways in which black women were excluded from the ability to protect their bodies, and the resulting civil discourse that has coalesced around taboo sexualities because of racism (see on the history of rape and the law Crenshaw 1989; Davis 1978; Hall 1983; Spillers 1984; for analysis of popular culture see hooks 1994). Moreover, the role and prominence of African American churches as the moral authority of black America is another factor that makes discussions of sexuality that is

not within the heterosexual monogamous realm difficult. Therefore, with the negation of black sexuality in the public sphere and the moral responsibility of "the race" often placed upon the shoulders of African American women, these constraints make it difficult for the rights of black prostitutes to be voiced and taken seriously. These ideas are all factors that I think have not been taken into consideration when thinking about the creation of public "sex worker identities."

CHAPTER TWO: WOMEN'S NARRATIVE BIO-SKETCHES

1. T-cells are the cells that govern immune system functioning. It is important for people with the HIV/AIDS virus to monitor the level of these cells because of their importance in the overall maintenance of the body.

2. Although Charlene indicated that crack was a significant problem in her life, her longest-standing addiction has been to alcohol. Interestingly enough, she never entered a treatment program for heroin or crack cocaine use.

3. This was a common occurrence among respondents.

4. Collins (1990) describes how U.S. society's emphasis on European centered ideals of beauty has had a negative impact on African American women.

5. Other respondents, such as Simone, cite similar problems. There are also women outside the deep sample who have experienced inter- and intraracial discrimination because of their skin color.

6. This is a popular term among respondents. The usage of the word suggests several meanings: (1) knowing about sexual topics at a young age; (2) pursuing sexual activity at a young age, or (3) trying to act "adultlike." Overall, the word constitutes a description for a range of behaviors and attitudes that are connected to sexuality. The term can have a positive, negative, or neutral meaning.

7. I have discovered from analyzing respondents' narratives (both inside and outside of the deep sample) that death of a loved one at an early age can trigger early substance use.

8. Billy Jean also feels she has let her family down because she has not properly fulfilled her "role" as a woman. This belief has extremely negative consequences on her ability to focus on her own life goals.

9. Later on she pursued and received her GED.

10. The term 151s refers to a rolled marijuana cigarette laced with powdered cocaine. There is some cross-cultural variation in the meanings of 151s. In some places 151s refer to cigars with marijuana and powdered cocaine rolled together (see Inciardi, Lockwood, and Potteigier 1993; Ratner 1993).

11. Cherise is the only self-identified lesbian in the deep sample.

12. If their partners introduced them to crack, many women (in the total sample) construct a "seduction of crack" narrative. I label their narratives this way because the women present themselves as innocent, helpless, and seduced both by their lovers and the drug. They will describe the drug and its effect on them in almost sensual terms. These portrayals of themselves as hapless people are often in direct contrast or conflict with other aspects of their narratives.

13. At the time of the research Detroit had few inpatient treatment programs for substance-using women who were also pregnant.

14. In many of my interviews, if a woman reported an estranged relationship with her mother, she frequently noted that pregnancy changed her status in the house. For example, if the woman had been responsible for the majority of the cooking and other household chores, she was released from these activities; her mother often pampered her. Respondents often felt ambivalent about the new attention they received and resentful after the child was born, when their regular status resumed.

15. The common terms used by respondents for men who purchase sex from women are "john" and "trick" or "client."

16. See the appendix

17. Early adultlike responsibility, which precluded them from enjoying their childhood, is a theme echoed in many respondents' stories, including those of Cynthia, Anna, Georgia, and Charlene.

18. This is also not an uncommon occurrence among respondents.

19. In another interview, Georgia talked candidly about the ruthlessness of street life. She discussed how it often presented poor choices for women. Her desire for independence and status within the world of the informal drug economy prompted her to partake in activities that she felt hurt other women, including helping her husband "pimp" other women.

Chapter Three: Capturing the Research Journey/ Listening to Women's Lives

1. Although Herron's argument is compelling, new events in Detroit's unfolding political history suggest Detroit might again be able to create political and social meaning for its citizens, and for the nation.

2. David M. Katzman (1973) provides a comprehensive overview of Detroit's early history and, specifically, of African Americans' struggle for racial and economic equality.

3. Although there is currently an intellectual renaissance in studying stigmatized populations, particularly sex workers (see Kempadoo and Doezema 1998; Chapkis 1997; Hoigard and Finstad 1986; Troung 1990), when I was graduate student there were few (inside or outside my home discipline of political science) I could turn to for help who had dealt with the difficulties and peculiarities of establishing a field presence or working with these populations.

4. See the appendix.

5. FIT Street Outreach wanted women to make better choices for themselves, but this did not necessarily mean leaving the street. They viewed sex work as a practice and a lifestyle that has traditionally disadvantaged women. But they did not espouse the idea that prostitution had to be abolished, nor did they ignore the complex reasons why women worked on the street.

6. I was asked not to interview anyone while I was on a shift nor approach anyone who was receiving services through FIT's programs.

7. I discuss some of the challenges of working at FIT, dealing with gatekeepers at various organizations, and gaining access to respondents; see Feldman, Bell, and Berger 2003.

8. See the appendix.

9. As the research progressed, I interviewed as many women as I could at the courthouse or nearby because I often found the phone numbers given to me were not reliable. Sometimes, I would wind up having to discuss why someone had not seen his or her daughter, cousin, sister, partner, and so forth in the last couple of days, months, or years.

10. In the field, I tried to keep the definition of sex work broad—as the exchange of sexual services for crack cocaine or other drugs, food, money, housing, clothing, and other material items. I found this definitional range to be helpful, because many of the women did exchange sexual services (in the broadest sense) for a large array of material items (in the broadest sense). Sex work could also include escort services, massage, phone sex, exotic dancing, and the like.

11. During this time I started developing frameworks about stigma, which would later comprise the concept of intersectional stigma, though I had not officially come up with the term.

12. See the appendix

13. I often thought of my other role in the field as a "resource person" to some of the women. For example, sometimes a woman turned to me for computer assistance or writing assistance or asked me to talk with her children about the benefits of staying in school. Being a resource person was important to me and most of the time did not drain my financial or emotional resources. This also built rapport with the respondents. Rapport is an important component in getting and sustaining access (see Feldman, Bell, and Berger 2003).

14. I sent the tapes to a transcriber, reviewed the transcripts for mistakes, and also took notes on my impressions of both the tapes and transcripts.

15. Sexuality is compounded in the field when one factors in the interrelated dimensions of race and ethnicity. Intersectional experiences of women of color researchers (anthropologists or other qualitative researchers) are scant (see Feldman, Bell, and Berger 2003; McClaurin 2001; Twine and Warren 2000). Given the social construction of sexuality for women of color, there are bound to be repercussions for the researcher in the field, especially if the topic is sexualized. Crenshaw (1989, 1997), Hammonds (1997) hooks (1981, 1984), Hurtado (1996), and Wallace (1992) all have developed sophisticated critiques concerning the representation of women of color's sexuality in dominant culture.

16. The idea of a woman addicted to crack who is a sexual "fiend" and uncontrollable has been an image and interpretation put forth through both academic and the popular media. Much of the ethnographic literature on women and crack cocaine use focuses on sex-for-crack exchanges (Inciardi 1993; Ratner 1993). The terms used to refer to women on the street are often derogatory and demeaning. Berger (1998), Jones (1992), and Wallace (1992) all provide detailed analyses of how black women have been represented in various popular movies of the eighties and nineties as crack cocaine users.

17. Notable exceptions to this phenomenon are Boyd and Gutherie 1996; Boyd 1993; Maher 1992, 1997 and Murphy and Rosenbaum 1995, who look at women's complex experiences using drugs.

18. I think this is a common fear when a researcher attempts to study a devalued group or population, whether one consciously admits it or not. Researchers are conditioned to find the "exciting" parts of a story (see Devault 1999). And, many of

the frames through which we typically view life and value life experiences have been criticized as androcentric (Smith 1987). For example, women's experiences of religion, politics, and work (to name broad areas of life experience) do not correspond to men's experiences, for a multitude of complex reasons. They are all areas which researchers are just beginning to explore and create new narratives about.

19. Postmodernists and others might take strong objection to the idea that there is an "honest voice" of women. I, however, take Anderson and Jack as suggesting that without approaching gender strategically in the interviewing process, we will reproduce what we already know of women's lives.

20. Transgender prostitutes (male to female) who wanted to be interviewed brought my assumptions about the category of "woman" to my attention in Detroit. At that point in time I stuck to interviewing "biological" females, and thus privileging one manifestation of "female identity." Knowing what I know today, I might have made several different choices along the way. Feinberg (1996) provides a broad history on transgender identity and its multiple meanings in society.

21. Although several of the women discussed troubling experiences that did easily fit into the "violence against women" rubric, they were more complicated than simple "male violence" against women.

Chapter Four: Narratives of Injustice: Discovery of the HIV/AIDS Virus

1. By early wave, I refer to the argument that concerning the HIV/AIDS virus, women's issues during the late eighties and early nineties were given little national medical and research attention (Stoller 1998). It could be argued that this overall low priority concerning women and HIV/AIDS contributes in part to explaining some of the women's negative and degrading experiences, as discussed in the latter half of the chapter.

2. The current procedure for getting an HIV/AIDS test consists of a person going to a designated testing facility and taking a blood test. Later the person goes to the testing facility to get the results.

3. Julianna had a newly born daughter, who when first tested for HIV/AIDS did not show signs of the HIV/AIDS virus. Often a baby will later test positive for the antibodies of HIV (also known as seroconversion) gotten through mother's milk or from other fluids while the child was in the womb.

4. This is also an example of theme two, Julianna receiving the message that death was imminent.

5. See the appendix.

6. See the appendix.

7. Her account brings up concerns about the medical and psychological treatment of female inmates.

8. See the appendix.

9. This is evidence of theme one.

10. See the appendix.

11. See the appendix.

12. Billy Jean's account also suggests that she too received little to no information and is evidence of theme one.

13. Julianna and Constance are both college-educated women and grew up in middle-income homes. They may not have had negative expectations of public health facilities.

14. Given Shelly's experiences with sexual and physical abuse by members of her community, these fears seem justified. Women's prior experience from being on the street also contributed to fears of retaliation because of their HIV-status. Women were often beaten, taunted, and raped because they were drug users and viewed as crack "fiends." Their drug-using status on the street was a tenuous one. People, especially men, perpetuated acts that could "teach them a lesson" about being a woman who used crack cocaine. Maher (1997) and Inciardi (1993) document the continuum of violence that women using crack cocaine routinely face. Jody Miller (1993, 1995) documents how women crack cocaine users try to resist and combat overt acts of violence and humiliation.

15. At the time Billy Jean was not sure of the child's paternal identity. She later went on to describe how periodically, the man (who did turn out to be the child's father) with whom she was staying with would alternate between asking her to have an abortion (because of his beliefs about HIV) and wanting her to have the child.

16. See the appendix.

17. Shenna's social status as a white woman was undercut through her history of sex work and drug use.

18. Unfortunately there have not been systematic studies that chronicle women's experiences with providers during the HIV testing and counseling process. I have found anecdotal material in various works on women and HIV that suggest many women—both stigmatized and nonstigmatized—have similar experiences (see Cuccinelli and De Groot 1997; Lather and Smithies 1997, chap. 5).

19. Battle also provides an interesting account of working with staff members who routinely made derogatory remarks to both HIV-positive and non-HIV-positive lower-income African American women.

20. Some would argue the research focus on pregnant women and HIV/AIDS reinforces the idea that women's health issues should primarily be linked to child-bearing (see Patton 1994; Schneider and Stoller 1995).

21. Nicole is discussing a documented phenomenon, that women with HIV, particularly women of color, often have gone undiagnosed by doctors. One author argues that "these women die as a result of opportunistic infections without ever having been considered for treatment eligibility" (Land 1994, 288).

CHAPTER FIVE: LIFE RECONSTRUCTION AND THE DEVELOPMENT OF NONTRADITIONAL POLITICAL RESOURCES

1. I discuss this point in the next chapter.

2. There is wide variation in treatment centers as to whether clients will receive individual counseling. Almost all treatment programs provide group counseling and ongoing support groups.

3. More research needs to be conducted on HIV-positive women who are also sexual survivors. Many of my respondents who were sexually abused felt that their abuse involved them in other high-risk activities at an early age.

CHAPTER SIX: LIFE RECONSTRUCTION AND GENDER

1. This is consistent with other research on female lawbreakers (see Maher 1997).

2. Women who were diagnosed prior to 1992 discussed that often when they told doctors of the types of symptoms they were experiencing in relation to the HIV/AIDS virus, their symptoms were dismissed.

3. Although current research on women who use crack (or other drugs) does not allow for the multiplicity of experiences of sex work, my research with women suggests more attention be given to these issues (see also Maher 1997; Pettigrew 1997).

4. I have chosen not to focus on the experiences of women who exchange sex for crack. I have done this because sex-for-crack exchanges were one of the least interesting features of the women's experiences. When discussing this feature of their addiction, women expressed shame, reservation, and regret. They did not express these things necessarily when generally talking about drug exchanges or sex work exchanges.

5. This idea is overwhelmingly consistent for the majority of the respondents in the total sample. The idea they are "driven" into prostitution and sex work because of drug use was simply not a useful reference point in analyzing this population of women's experiences. Again, experiences with sex work for many respondents included being a call girl, walking the street, nude modeling, stripping, working in bars or hotels, often before any serious or addictive drug use.

6. This is less the case with people like Cynthia, Daria, and Kitt, who express conflicting ideas about their sex work histories. All of them share molestation in their childhood background. The linkage between sex work and childhood molestation has been a debated issue (see Barry 1995). Despite what conclusions we might want to draw from the research on this topic, the women here assume a relatively nonbiased opinion about sex work, especially with the women whom they come into contact with through their community work.

7. See the appendix.

8. This quote is highlighted again for different reasons in chapter 7.

9. Some women have opted to date HIV-positive men they might meet through their HIV/AIDS work, jobs, and social contacts. Even if they decided to pursue liaisons with HIV-positive men, they realized they had to assume responsibility for their own health.

10. I want to stress the importance of deciding to live with HIV/AIDS. During the early stages of HIV, many of the women wanted to or did try to commit suicide (consciously or unconsciously through the heavy use of drugs). The decision to live is a conscious one among respondents.

11. There are other accounts of women with HIV who use this term of "being a women with HIV." The accounts are anecdotal and I have not seen this linked to further politicization, but it definitely connotes a point in a person's life where they are comfortable with living with the disease. Lather and Smithies (1997) discussion of their work with HIV-positive women in support groups is relevant here.

12. In the overall sample, women typically described themselves as loners. A common response was from Joyce, a twenty-three-year-old African American

woman who is HIV-negative in the larger sample. She has been in treatment twice:

> MICHELE: *Do you get along with women on the street*
> JOYCE: *No! I fight with them.*

13. See the appendix.

CHAPTER SEVEN: MAKING WORKABLE SISTERHOOD POSSIBLE

1. Of those looking at different populations both Boehmer (2000) and Naples (1991b) discuss similar findings from their ethnographic work on women and activism.

2. There are a few people in the deep sample about which this observation does not apply. For example, Julianna's mother was incredibly active in community politics while Julianna was growing up. The majority of the women, however, voted for the first time after becoming HIV-positive. Given that many of the women were already involved by their early twenties in numerous types of law-breaking and stigmatizing activities, these conditions alone would tend to circumscribe or preclude their interest and ability to engage in political participation.

3. Women often discussed their ideas about politics and inequality in the same context of their parent's negative experiences either in the workplace (because of discrimination) or in society in general.

4. There is a well-developed literature in political science that discusses the extent to which blacks in particular feel less efficacious in participating in public institutions (see Cohen 1999). Rosenstone and Hansen (1993) have written extensively about the importance of resources for effective participation.

5. McBride (1991) discusses the role of epidemics as experienced by urban blacks, and how the history of government mismanagement and neglect has shaped African American's perspectives of epidemics. James Jones (1981) documents the Tuskegee syphilis experiments on African American men. Cohen (1993) discusses the impact of these experiences as shaping collective thought in African American communities: For instance, community members do not have to reach far back into their collective memory to recall the racist blame placed on the community for the origin of other diseases such as tuberculosis and syphilis. Further ingrained in the minds of black Americans is the medical exploitation of black sharecroppers during the Tuskegee syphilis experiments. And not long ago stories developed claiming Africa, in particular the "green monkey" in Africa, to be the source of AIDS (Cohen 1993, 82).

6. This will become clearer through a discussion of Constance's experiences in the medical arena. Respondents' experiences and the experiences of the people they serve constantly reinforce their opinion that the medical community, in particular, does not provide them with adequate services. Stoller (1998) cites evidence that medical providers and medical staff have been uncomfortable providing services to current and former drug users who have HIV.

7. This is particularly true of the women who concentrate on HIV-positive women's services.

8. See the appendix.

9. Sometimes agencies have resources to provide a very small amount of money for the role of advocate that is a volunteer position.

10. See the appendix

11. Nicole is the only woman to have kept strong ties with the Detroit Department of Health.

12. Although it is not discussed in this chapter, Constance had expressed similar concerns about the HIV-positive substance users.

13. Recall Julianna's experience with the Department of Health in chapter 4.

14. See the appendix.

15. See the appendix.

16. A distinction needs to be made here. There are several programs run through city agencies throughout Detroit that have provided services for people with HIV; these programs are not usually run by HIV-positive people, which is often a sticking point for many of the respondents.

17. I was told by another source that some women in the local HIV/AIDS community who did not know me called Constance to find out about this "young woman researcher" who was asking questions about women and HIV.

18. See the appendix.

19. Inglewood is a fictitious name for a large suburban community near Metro Detroit, where Shenna grew up.

20. Keith Haring was an openly gay man who used a combination of graffiti and modern arts techniques to develop art that was community inspired and addressed social issues. His work inspired a generation of artists in the eighties. He died of AIDS in 1990.

21. This term was popularized by Alice Walker (1983) and is a term that locates African American women and other women of color's struggles against *gendered racism* and exploitation within a legacy of resistance.

Bibliography

Abu-Lughod, L. 1988. "Fieldwork of a Dutiful Daughter." In *Studying Your Own Society: Arab Women in the Field*, edited by S. Altorki and C. El-Solh, 139–61. Syracuse, N.Y.: Syracuse University Press.

Ackelsberg, Martha. 1988. "Communities, Resistance, and Women's Activism: Some Implications for a Democratic Polity." In *Women and the Politics of Empowerment*, edited by Ann Bookman and Sandra Morgen, 297–313. Philadelphia: Temple University Press.

ACT UP/New York Women and AIDS Book Group. 1992. *Women, AIDS, and Activism*. Boston: South End Press.

Ainlay, Stephen C., Gaylene Becker, and Lerita Coleman, eds. 1986. *The Dilemma of Difference: A Multidisciplinary View of Stigma*. New York: Plenum Press.

———. 1986. "Stigma Reconsidered." In *The Dilemma of Difference: A Multidisciplinary View of Stigma*, edited by Stephen Ainlay, Gaylene Becker, and Lerita Coleman. New York, 1–13. Plenum Press.

Alexander, Priscilla. 1995. "Sex Workers Fight against AIDS: An International Perspective." In *Women Resisting AIDS: Feminist Strategies of Empowerment*, edited by Beth E. Schneider and Nancy E. Stoller, 99–123. Philadelphia: Temple University Press.

Alonzo, Angelo, and Nancy Reynolds. 1995. "Stigma, HIV, and AIDS: An Exploration and Elaboration of a Stigma Trajectory." *Social Science and Medicine* 41, no. 3 (August): 303–15.

Amaro, Hortensia. 1995. "Love, Sex, and Power: Considering Women's Realities in HIV Prevention—Award Address." *American Psychologist* 50, no. 6 (June): 437–47.

American Medical Association. 2001. "Report on Racial and Ethnic Disparities in Health Care." Washington, D.C.: American Medical Association.

Andersen, Margaret, and Patricia Hill Collins, eds. 1992. *Race, Class, and Gender: An Anthology*. Belmont, Calif.: Wadsworth Publishing.

Anderson, Elijah. 1990. *Streetwise: Race, Class, and Change in an Urban Community*. Chicago: University of Chicago Press.

Anderson, Kathryn, and Dana C. Jack. 1991. "Learning to Listen: Interview Techniques and Analyses." In *Women's Words: The Feminist Practice of Oral History*, edited by Sherna B. Gluck and Daphne Patai, 11–26. New York: Routledge.

Anzandula, Gloria, and Cherrie Moraga, eds. 1990. *Making Face/Making Soul*. New York: Kitchen Table Press.

Arnold, Regina. 1990. "Processes of Victimization and Criminalization of Black Women." *Social Justice* 17, no. 3: 153–66.

Austin, Regina. 1992a. " 'The Black Community,' Its Lawbreakers, and a Politics of Identification." *Southern California Law Review* 65, no. 2 (May): 1769–1817.

Austin, Regina. 1992b. "Black Women, Sisterhood, and the Difference/Deviance Divide." *New England Law Review* 26, no.14: 877–87.

———. 1989. Sapphire Bound! *Wisconsin Law Review* 54, no. 8: 539–78.

Bambara, Toni Cade. 1980. *The Salt Eaters*. New York: Vintage.

Barnard, C. P. 1989. "Alcoholism and Sex Abuse in the Family: Incest and Marital Rape." *Journal of Chemical Dependency Treatment* 3:131–44.

Barry, Kathleen. 1995. *The Prostitution of Sexuality*. New York: New York University Press.

Battle, Shelia. 1997. "The Bond Is Called Blackness: Black Women and AIDS." In *The Gender Politics of HIV/AIDS in Women*, edited by Nancy Goldstein and Jennifer Manlowe, 282–92. New York: New York University Press.

Beale, Frances. 1970. "Double Jeopardy: To Be Black and Female." In *The Black Woman*, edited by Toni Cade Bambara, 90–100. New York: New American Library.

Becker, Gaylene, and Regina Arnold. 1986. "Stigma as a Cultural Construct." In *The Dilemma of Difference: A Multidisciplinary View of Stigma*, edited by Stephen Ainlay, Gaylene Becker, and Lerita Coleman, 39–55. New York: Plenum Press.

Becker, Howard S. 1963. *Outsiders*. New York: Free Press.

Behar, Ruth. 1993. *Translated Woman: Crossing the Border with Esperanza's Story*. Boston: Beacon Press.

Belenky, Mary, Blythe McVicker Clinchy, Nancy Rule Goldberger, and Jill Mattuck Tarule. 1997. *Women's Ways of Knowing: The Development of Self, Voice, and Mind*. 2d ed. New York: Basic Books.

Bell, Laurie, ed. 1987. *Good Girls/Bad Girls: Feminists and Sex Trade Workers Face to Face*. Toronto: Seal Press.

Bell, Shannon. 1994. *Reading, Writing, and Rewriting the Prostitute Body*. Bloomington: Indiana University Press.

Bennett, M. 1990. "Stigmatization: Experiences of Persons with Acquired Immune Deficiency Syndrome." *Issues in Mental Health Nursing* 1, no. 18: 141–45.

Berger, Michele. 1998. HomeGirls and Skeezers: Representations of Crack and Prostitution. Paper presented at the conference of the National Women's Studies Association.

Boehmer, Ulrike. 2000. *The Personal and the Political: Women's Activism in Response to the Breast Cancer and AIDS Epidemics*. Albany: State University of New York Press.

Bookman, Ann, and Sandra Morgen. 1988. "'Carry It On': Continuing the Discussion and the Struggle." In *Women and the Politics of Empowerment*, edited by Ann Bookman and Sandra Morgen, 314–22. Philadelphia: Temple University Press.

Borland, Katherine. 1991. "'That's Not What I Said': Interpretative Conflict in Oral Narrative Research." In *Women's Words: The Feminist Practice of Oral History*, edited by Sherna B. Gluck and Daphne Patai, 63–75. New York: Routledge.

Bourgois, Phillippe, and Eloise Dunlap. 1993. "Exorcising Sex-for-Crack: An Ethnographic Perspective from Harlem." In *Crack Pipe as Pimp*, edited by Mitchell S. Ratner, 97–132. New York: Lexington Books.

Boyd, Carol. 1993. "The Antecedents of Women's Crack Cocaine Abuse: Family Substance Abuse, Sexual Abuse, Depression, and Illicit Drug Use." *Journal of Substance Abuse Treatment* 10:433–38.

Boyd, Carol, Fredric Blow, and Linda S. Orgain. 1993. "Gender Differences among African-American Substance Abusers." *Journal of Psychoactive Drugs* 25, no. 4: 301–5.

Boyd, Carol, and Barbara Gutherie. 1996. "Women, Their Significant Others, and Crack Cocaine." *American Journal on Addictions* 5, no. 2 (Spring): 156–66.

Boyd, Carol, Barbara Gutherie, Joanne Pohl, Jason Whitemarsh, and Dorothy Henderson. 1994. "African-American Women Who Smoke Crack Cocaine: Sexual Trauma and the Mother-Daughter Relationship." *Journal of Psychoactive Drugs* 26, no. 3 (September–October): 243–47.

Brandt, Allan. 1985. *No Magic Bullet: A Social History of Venereal Disease in the United States since 1880*. New York: Oxford University Press.

Brewer, Rose M. 1993. "Theorizing Race, Class, and Gender: The New Scholarship of Black Feminist Intellectuals and Black Women's Labor." In *Theorizing Black Feminisms*, edited by S. James and A. Busia, 13–30. New York: Routledge.

Burgess, Robert G. 1982. *Field Research: A Sourcebook and Field Manual*. London: George Allen and Unwin.

Butler, Judith. 1990. *Gender Trouble*. New York: Routledge.

Butler, Judith, and Joan W. Scott, eds. 1992. *Feminists Theorize the Political*. New York: Routledge.

Cannon, Katie. 1985. "The Emergence of Black Feminist Consciousness." In *Feminist Interpretation of the Bible*, edited by Letty M. Russell, 30–40. Philadelphia: Westminister.

Campbell, Nancy. 2000. *Using Women: Gender, Drug Policy, and Social Justice*. New York: Routledge.

Carlomusto, Jean. 1992. "Focusing on Women: Videos as Activism." In *Women, AIDS, and Activism*, edited by ACT UP/New York Women and AIDS Book Group, 215–18. Boston: South End Press.

Cash, Kathlee. 1996. "Women Educating Women for HIV/AIDS Prevention." In *Women's Experiences with HIV/AIDS: An International Experience*, edited by Lynellyn Long and E. Maxine Ankrah, 311–32. New York: Columbia University Press.

Chancer, Lynn Sharon. 1993. "Prostitution, Feminist Theory, and Ambivalence: Notes from the Sociological Underground." *Social Text* 11, no. 4 (Winter): 143–71.

Chapkis, Wendy. 1997. *Live Sex Acts: Women Performing Erotic Labor*. New York: Routledge.

Charlton, James I. 1998. *Nothing about Us without Us: Disability Oppression and Empowerment*. Berkeley and Los Angeles: University of California Press.

Chasnoff, Ira J. 1990. "The Prevalence of Illicit Drug or Alcohol Use during Pregnancy and Discrepancies in Mandatory Reporting in Pinellas County, Florida." *New England Journal of Medicine* 322: 1201–6.

Chavkin, Wendy. 1991. "Mandatory Treatment for Drug Use during Pregnancy." *Journal of the American Medical Association* 266 (September): 1556–61.

Chow, Ester Ngan-lin, Doris Wilkerson, and Maxine Baca Zinn, eds. 1996. *Race, Class, and Gender: Common Bonds, Different Voices*. Thousand Oaks, Calif.: Sage Publications.

Christensen, Kim. 1992. "How Do Women Live?" In *Women, AIDS, and Activism*, edited by ACT UP/New York Women and AIDS Book Group, 5–15. Boston: South End Press.

Chu, S. Y., J. Buehler, and R. Berkelman. 1990. "Impact of the Human Immuno-deficiency Virus Epidemic on Mortality in Women of Reproductive Age, United States." *Journal of the American Medical Association* 264 (July): 225–29.

Clifford, James, and George E. Marcus, eds. 1986. *The Poetics and Politics of Ethnography*. Berkeley and Los Angeles: University of California Press.

Cohen, Cathy. 1999. *The Boundaries of Blackness: AIDS and the Breakdown of Black Politics*. Chicago: University of Chicago Press.

———. 1997. "Introduction: Women Transforming U.S. Politics: Sites of Power/Resistance." In *Women Transforming Politics: An Alternative Reader*, edited by Cathy Cohen, Kathleen B. Jones, and Joan C. Tronto, 1–14. New York: New York University Press.

———. 1993. Power, Resistance, and the Construction of Crisis: Marginalized Communities Respond to AIDS. Ph.D. dissertation. University of Michigan.

Cohen, Cathy, Kathleen B. Jones, and Joan C. Tronto, eds. 1997. *Women Transforming Politics: An Alternative Reader*. New York: New York University Press.

Collins, Patricia Hill. 1995. "Symposium on West and Fenstermaker's 'Doing Difference.'" *Gender and Society* 9, no. 4 (August): 491–94.

———. 1990. *Black Feminist Thought*. Boston: Unwin Hyman.

Combahee River Collective. 1979. "A Black Feminist Statement." In *But Some of Us Are Brave: Black Women's Studies*, edited by Gloria T. Hull, Patricia Bell Scott, and Barbara Smith, 13–22. New York: Monthly Review Press.

Cott, Nancy. 1987. *The Grounding of Modern Feminism*. New Haven: Yale University Press.

Crenshaw, Kimberle. 1997. "Beyond Racism and Misogyny: Black Feminisms and 2 Live Crew." In *Women Transforming Politics: An Alternative Reader*, edited by Cathy Cohen, Kathleen B. Jones, and Joan C. Tronto, 549–68. New York: New York University Press.

———. 1989. "Demarginalizing the Intersection of Race and Sex: A Black Feminist Critique of Antidiscrimination Doctrine, Feminist Theory, and Antiracist Politics." *University of Chicago Legal Forum* 139, no. 3: 139–67.

Cuccinelli, Debi, and Anne S. De Groot. 1997. "Put Her in a Cage: Childhood Sexual Abuse, Incarceration, and HIV Infection." In *The Gender Politics of HIV/AIDS in Women*, edited by Nancy Goldstein and Jennifer Manlowe, 222–41. New York: New York University Press.

Daly, Kathleen. 1993. "Class-Race-Gender: Sloganeering in Search of Meaning." *Social Justice* 20:56–71.

Daly, Kathleen, and Deborah J. Stephens. 1994. "The 'Dark Figure' of Criminology: Toward a black and Multi-ethnic Feminist Agenda for Theory and Research." Unpublished manuscript on file with the author.

Davis, Angela. 2003. *Are Prisons Obsolete?* New York: Seven Stories Press.

———. 1989. *Women, Culture, and Politics*. New York: Random House.

———. 1981. *Women, Race, and Class*. New York: Random House.

———. 1978. "Rape, Racism and the Capitalist Setting." *Black Scholar* 9, no. 7 (June): 24–30.

Dent, Gina, ed. 1992. *Black Popular Culture*. Seattle: Bay Press.

Delacoste, Fredrique, and Priscilla Alexander, eds. 1987. *Sex Work: Writings by Women in the Sex Industry*. Pittsburgh: Cleis Press.

Denison, Rebecca. 1995. "Call Us Survivors! Women Organized to Respond to Life Threatening Diseases (WORLD)." In *Women Resisting AIDS: Feminist Strategies of Empowerment*, edited by Beth E. Schneider and Nancy Stoller, 195–207. Philadelphia: Temple University Press.

Devault, Marjorie L. 1999. *Liberating Method: Feminism and Social Research*. Philadelphia: Temple University Press.

———. 1990. "Talking and Listening from Women's Standpoint: Feminist Strategies for Interviewing and Analysis." *Social Problems* 37 (February): 96–116.

De Zalduondo, Barbara. 1991. "Prostitution Viewed Cross-Culturally: Toward Recontextualizing Sex Work in AIDS Intervention Research." *Journal of Sex Research* 28, no. 2 (May): 223–48.

DiAna, DiAna. 1992. "Talking that Talk." In *Women, AIDS, and Activism*, edited by ACT UP/New York Women and AIDS Book Group, 219–22. Boston: South End Press.

Diaz, E. 1991. "Public Policy, Women, and HIV Disease." *SIECUS Report* 19 no. 2 (January): 4–5.

Dill, Bonnie Thorton. 1983. "Race, Class, and Gender: Prospects for an All-Inclusive Sisterhood." *Feminist Studies* 9, no.1 (Spring): 131–50.

———. 1979. "The Dialectics of Black Womanhood." *Signs* 4, no. 3: 543–55.

Dixon, Dazon. 1992. "Facing Reality: AIDS Education and Women of Color." In *Women, AIDS and Activism*, edited by ACT UP/New York Women and AIDS Book Group, 227–29. Boston: South End Press.

Douglas, Susan, J. 1994. *Where the Girls Are: Growing Up Female in the Mass Media*. New York: Times Books.

Downing, Moher. 1995. "Some Comments on the Beginnings of AIDS Outreach to Women Drug Users in San Francisco." In *Women Resisting AIDS: Feminist Strategies to Empowerment*, edited by Beth E. Schneider and Nancy Stoller, 231–45. Philadelphia: Temple University Press.

Dunlap, Eloise. 1992. "The Impact of Drugs on Family Life and Kin Networks in the Inner City African-American Single Parent Household." In *Drugs, Crime, and Social Isolation*, edited by Adele V. Harrell and George E. Peterson, 181–208. Washington, D.C.: Urban Institute Press.

Dworkin, Andrea. 1987. *Intercourse*. New York: Free Press.

Easton, David, and Jack Dennis. 1969. *Children and the Political System*. New York: McGraw-Hill.

Ehrenreich, Barbara, and Deidre English. 1973. *Complaints and Disorders: The Sexual Politics of Sickness*. New York: Vintage.

Epstein, Steven. 1991. "Democratic Science? AIDS Activism and the Contested Construction of Knowledge." *Socialist Review* 21, no. 2 (April–June): 33–50.

Esu-Williams, Eka. 1995. "AIDS in the 1990s: Individual and Collective Responsibility." In *Women Resisting AIDS: Feminist Strategies of Empowerment*, edited by Beth E. Schneider and Nancy Stoller, 23–31. Philadelphia: Temple University Press.

Evans, S., and S. Schaefer. 1980. "Why Women's Sexuality Is Important to Address in Chemical Dependency Programs." *Grassroots* 37:37–40.

Feinberg, Leslie. 1996. *Transgender Warriors: Making History from Joan of Arc to Dennis Rodman*. Boston: Beacon Press.

Feldman, Harvey, Frank Espanda, Sharon Penn, and Sharon Byrd. 1993. "Street Status and the Sex-for-Crack Scene in San Francisco." In *Crack Pipe as Pimp*, edited by Mitchell S. Ratner, 133–58. New York: Lexington Books.

Feldman, Martha, Jeannine Bell, and Michele Berger, eds. 2003. *Gaining Access: A Practical and Theoretical Guide for Qualitative Researchers*. Walnut Creek, Calif.: AltaMira Press.

Flammang, Janet A. 1997. *Women's Political Voice: How Women Are Transforming the Practice and Study of Politics*. Philadelphia: Temple University Press.

Flaskerud, Jacqueline H., and Adeline M. Nyamathi. 1990. "Effects of an AIDS Education Program on the Knowledge, Attitudes, and Practices of Low Income Black and Latina Women." *Journal of Community Health* 15, no. 6 (December): 343–55.

Forney, Mary, James Inciardi, and Dorothy Lockwood. 1992. "Exchanging Sex For Crack Cocaine: A Comparison of Women from Rural and Urban Communities." *Journal of Community Health* 17, no. 2: 73–85.

Foucault, Michel. *Discipline and Punish: The Birth of the Prison*. New York: Vintage Books, 1979.

Fraser, Marcy, and Diane Jones. 1995. "The Role of Nurses in the HIV Epidemic." In *Women Resisting AIDS: Feminist Strategies of Empowerment*, edited by Beth E. Schneider and Nancy Stoller, 286–98. Philadelphia: Temple University Press.

Friedman, Jennifer, and Marisa Alicea. 2001. *Surviving Heroin: Interviews with Women in Methadone Clinics*. Gainesville: University of Florida Press.

French, John F. 1993. "Pipe Dreams: Crack and the Life of Philadelphia and Newark." In *Crack Pipe as Pimp*, edited by Mitchell S. Ratner, 205–32. New York: Lexington Books.

Fulenwider, Claire Knoche. 1985. "Feminist Ideology, and the Political Attitudes and Participation of White and Minority Women." *Western Political Quarterly* 34 (March): 17–30.

Fullilove, Mindy, Robert E. Fullilove, Katherine Haynes, and Shirley Gross. 1990. "Black Women and AIDS Prevention: A View toward Understanding the Gender Rules." *Journal of Sex Research* 27 (February): 47–64.

Fullilove, Mindy, Anne Lown, and Robert Fullilove. 1992. "Crack 'Hos and Skeezers: Traumatic Experiences of Women Crack Users." *Journal of Sex Research* 29 (May): 275–87.

Fuss, Diana. 1989. *Essentially Speaking: Feminism, Nature, and Difference*. New York: Routledge.

Gaventa, John. 1980. *Power and Powerlessness: Quiescence and Rebellion in an Appalachian Valley*. Urbana: University of Illinois Press.

Geertz, Clifford. 1983. *Local Knowledge: Essays in Interpretive Anthropology*. New York: Basic Books.

———. 1973. *The Interpretation of Cultures*. New York: Basic Books.

Giddings, Paula. 1984. *When and Where I Enter: The Impact of Black Women on Race and Sex in America*. New York: William Morrow.

Gilkes, Cheryl Townsend. 1994. "'If It Wasn't for the Women . . .': African-American Women, Community Work, and Social Change." In *Women of Color in U.S. Society*, edited by Maxine Baca Zinn and Bonnie Thorton Dill. Philadelphia: Temple University Press.

———. 1990. "'Liberated to Work Like Dogs': Labeling Black Women and Their Work." In *The Experience and Meaning of Work in Women's Lives*, edited by Hildreth Y. Grossman and Nia Lane Chester. Hillsdale, N.J.: Lawrence Earlbaum Associates.

———. 1988. "Building in Many Places: Multiple Commitments and Ideologies on Black Women's Community Work." In *Women and The Politics of Empowerment*, edited by Ann Bookman and Sandra Morgen, 53–76. Philadelphia: Temple University Press.

———. 1983. "Going Up for the Oppressed: The Career Mobility of Black Women Community Workers." *Journal of Social Issues* 39, no. 3: 115–39.

———. 1980. "'Holding Back the Ocean with A Broom': Black Women and Community Work." In *The Black Woman*, edited by La Frances Rodgers-Rose, 217–31. Beverly Hills, Calif.: Sage Publications.

Gilligan, Carol. 1982. *In a Different Voice: Psychological Theory and Women's Development*. Cambridge: Harvard University Press.

Gilmore, Norbert, and Margaret A. Sommerville. 1994. "Stigmatization, Scapegoating and Discrimination in Sexually Transmitted Diseases: Overcoming 'Them' and Us." *Social Science and Medicine* 39, no. 9: 1339–58.

Glaser, Barney G., and Anslem L. Strauss. 1967. *The Discovery of Grounded Theory*. New York: Aldine De Gruyer.

Glover, Noreen M. 1999. "Play Therapy and Art Therapy for Substance Abuse Clients Who Have a History of Incest Victimization." *Journal of Substance Abuse Treatment* 16, no. 4 (June): 281–87.

Gluck, Sherna Berger, and Daphne Patai, eds. 1991. *Women's Words: The Feminist Practice of Oral History*. New York: Routledge.

Goffman, Erving. 1989. "On Fieldwork." *Journal of Contemporary Ethnography* 18 (July): 123–32.

———. 1971. *Stigma: Notes on the Management of Spoiled Identity*. Englewood Cliffs, N.J.: Prentice-Hall.

———. 1959. *The Presentation of Self in Everyday Life*. New York: Doubleday.

Goldstein, Nancy, and Jennifer Manlowe, eds. 1997. *The Gender Politics of HIV/AIDS in Women: Perspectives on the Pandemic in the United States*. New York: New York University Press.

Green, Gill. 1996. "Stigma and Social Relationships of People with HIV: Does Gender Make a Difference?" In *AIDS as a Gender Issue: Psychosocial Perspectives*, edited by Lorraine Sherr, Catherine Hankins, and Lydia Bennett, 46–63. London: Taylor and Francis.

Greenblat, Cathy Stein. 1995. "Women in Families with Hemophilia and HIV: Improving Communication about Sensitive Issues." In *Women Resisting AIDS: Feminist Strategies of Empowerment*, edited by Beth E. Schneider and Nancy E. Stoller, 124–38. Philadelphia: Temple University Press.

Grove, Kathleen A., Donald P. Kelly, and Judith Liu. 1997. "'But Nice Girls Don't Get It': Women, Symbolic Capital, and the Social Construction of AIDS." *Journal of Contemporary Ethnography* 26, no. 3: 317–37.

Gupta, Geeta Rao, Ellen Weiss, and Purnima Mane. 1996. "Talking about Sex: A Prerequisite for AIDS Prevention." In *Women's Experiences with HIV/AIDS: An International Perspective*, edited by Lynellyn Long and E. Maxine Ankrah, 333–50. New York: Columbia University Press.

Guralnik, David B., ed. 1982. *Webster's New World Dictionary*. New York: Simon and Schuster.

Hall, Jacqueline Dowd. 1983. "'The Mind That Burns in Each Body': Women, Rape, and Racial Violence." In *Powers of Desire: The Politics of Sexuality*, edited by Ann Snitow, Christine Stansell, and Sharon Thompson, 328–49. New York: Monthly Review Press.

Hammersely, Martin, and Peter Atkinson. 1983. *Ethnography: Principles in Practice*. London: Tavistock.

Hammonds, Evelynn M. 1997. "Seeing AIDS: Race, Gender, and Representation." In *The Gender Politics of HIV/AIDS in Women*, edited by Nancy Goldstein and Jennifer Manlowe, 113–26. New York: New York University Press.

Haraway, Donna. 1988. "Situated Knowledges: The Science Question in Feminism and the Privilege of Partial Perspective." *Feminist Studies* 14, no. 3: 575–99.

Hardcastle, David A., Stanley Wenocur, and Patricia Powers. 1997. *Community Practice: Theories and Skills for Social Workers*. London: Oxford University Press.

Harding, Sandra. 1986. *The Science Question in Feminism*. Ithaca: Cornell University Press.

Harris, Gail. 1992. "Changing the Whole Approach." In *Women, AIDS and Activism*, edited by ACT UP/New York Women and AIDS Book Group, 231–32. Boston: South End Press.

Hemphill, Essex, ed. 1991. *Brother to Brother: New Writings by Black Gay Men*. Boston: Alyson Publications.

Henslin, James, ed. 1995. *Down to Earth Sociology*. New York: Free Press.

Herek, Gregory M., John P. Capitanio, and Keith F. Widaman. 2002. "HIV-Related Stigma and Knowledge in the United States: Prevalence and Trends, 1991–1999." *American Journal of Public Health* 92, no.3 (March 2002): 371–77.

Herek, Gregory M., and John Capitanio. 1993. "Public Reactions to AIDS in the United States: A Second Decade of Stigma." *American Journal of Public Health*. 83, no. 4 (April): 574–77.

Herek, Gregory M., and Edward Glunt. 1988. "An Epidemic of Stigma: Public Reactions to AIDS." *American Psychologist* 5, no. 14: 886–93.

Herron, Jerry. 1993. *AfterCulture: Detroit and the Humiliation of History*. Detroit: Wayne State University Press.

Higginbotham, Evelyn. 1992. "African-American Women's History and the Metalanguage of Race." *Signs: Journal of Women in Culture and Society* 17 (Winter): 251–74.

Hobson, B. M. *Uneasy Virtue: The Politics of Prostitution: The American Reform Movement*. Chicago: University of Chicago Press, 1990.

Hoigard, Celie, and Liv Finstad. 1986. *Backstreets: Prostitution, Money, and Love*. University Park: Pennsylvania State University Press.

Hollibaugh, Amber. 1995. "Lesbian Denial and Lesbian Leadership in the AIDS Epidemic: Bravery and Fear in the Construction of a Lesbian Geography of Risk." In *Women Resisting AIDS: Feminist Strategies of Empowerment*, edited by Beth E. Schneider and Nancy Stoller, 219–30. Philadelphia: Temple University Press.

hooks, bell. 1994. *Outlaw Culture*. New York: Routledge.

———. 1989. *Talking Back: Thinking Feminist, Thinking Black*. Boston: South End Press.

———. 1984. *From Margin to Center*. Boston: South End Press.

———. 1981. *Ain't I a Woman: Black Women and Feminism*. Boston: South End Press.

Hughes, Everett Cherrington. 1945. "Dilemmas and Contradictions of Status." *American Journal of Sociology* 50 (March): 353–59.

Hurtado, Aida. 1989. "Relating to White Privilege: Seduction and Rejection in the Subordination of White Women and Women of Color." *Signs: Journal of Women in Culture and Society* 14 (Summer): 833–55.

Inciardi, James. 1993. "Kingrats, Chicken Heads, Slow Necks, Freaks, and Blood Suckers: A Glimpse at the Miami Sex for Crack Market." In *Crack Pipe as Pimp*, edited by Mitchell S. Ratner, 37–68. New York: Lexington Books.

Inciardi, James, Dorothy Lockwood, and Anne Potteigier. 1993. *Women and Crack Cocaine*. New York: Macmillan.

James, Joy, and Ruth Farmer, eds. 1993. *Spirit, Space, and Survival: African American Women in (White) Academe*. New York: Routledge.

Jenness, Valerie. 1993. *Making It Work: The Prostitute's Rights Movement in Perspective*. New York: Aldine de Gruyter.

Jones, Jacquie. 1992. "The Accusatory Space." In *Black Popular Culture*, edited by Gina Dent, 94–7. Seattle: Bay Press.

Jones, James H. 1981. *Bad Blood: The Tuskegee Syphilis Experiment: A Tragedy of Race and Medicine*. New York: Free Press.

Kalichman, S., J. Kelly, T. Hunter, D. Murphy, and R. Tyler. 1992. "Culturally Tailored HIV-AIDS Risk-Reduction Messages Targeted to African-American Urban Women: Impact on Risk Sensitization and Risk Reduction. *Journal of Counseling and Clinical Psychology*, 61:291–95.

Katzman, David M. 1973. *Before the Ghetto: Black Detroit in the Nineteenth Century*. Urbana: University of Illinois Press.

Kelley, Robin D. G. 1994. "Introduction: Writing Black Working-Class History from Way, Way Below." In *Race Rebels*, 1–16. New York: Free Press.

Kelly, Jacqueline A., Syrius St. Lawrence, Susan Smith, Vonda Hood, and D. Cook. 1987. "Stigmatization of AIDS Patients by Physicians." *American Journal of Public Health* 77:798–99.

Kempadoo, Kamala, and Jo Doezema, eds. 1998. *Global Sex Workers: Rights, Resistance, and Rebellion*. New York: Routledge.

King, Deborah K. 1988. "Multiple Jeopardy, Multiple Consciousness: The Context of a Black Feminist Ideology." *Signs: Journal of Women in Culture and Society* 14 (Autumn): 42–72.

Krauss, Celene. 1998. "Toxic Waste Protests and the Politicization of White, Working-Class Women." In *Community Activism and Feminist Politics: Organizing across Race, Class, and Gender*, edited by Nancy Naples, 129–50. New York: Routledge.

Land, Helen. 1994. "AIDS and Women of Color." *Families in Society: The Journal of Contemporary Human Services* 75 (June): 355–61.

Lather, Patti, and Chris Smithies. 1997. *Troubling the Angels: Women Living with HIV/AIDS*. Boulder, Colo.: Westview Press.

Lawless, Sonia, Susan Kippax, and June Crawford. 1996. "Dirty, Diseased, and Undeserving: The Positioning of HIV Positive Women." *Social Science and Medicine* 43, no. 9: 1371–77.

Leigh, Carol. 1997. "Inventing Sex Work." In *Whores and Other Feminists*, edited by Jill Nagle, 223–27. New York: Routledge.

Lewis, Diane K. 1995. "African-American Women at Risk: Notes on the Sociocultural Context of HIV Infection." In *Women Resisting AIDS: Feminist Strategies of Empowerment*, edited by Beth E. Schneider and Nancy Stoller, 57–73. Philadelphia: Temple University Press.

Lockett, Gloria. 1995. "Cal-PEP: The Struggle to Survive." In *Women Resisting AIDS: Feminist Strategies of Empowerment*, edited by Beth E. Schneider and Nancy Stoller, 208–18. Philadelphia: Temple University Press.

Long, Lynellyn. 1996. "Introduction: Counting Women's Experiences." In *Women's Experiences with HIV/AIDS: An International Perspective*, edited by Lynellyn Long and E. Maxine Ankrah, 1–22. New York: Columbia University Press.

Long, Lynellyn, and E. Maxine Ankrah, eds. 1996. *Women's Experiences with HIV/AIDS: An International Perspective*. New York: Columbia University Press.

Lorde, Audre. 1984. *Sister Outsider*. Trumansberg, N.Y.: Crossing Press.

Lubiano, Wahneena. 1993. "Black Ladies, Welfare Queens, and State Minstrels: Ideological Warfare by Narrative Means." In *Race-ing Justice, En-Gendering Power: Essays on Anita Hill, Clarence Thomas, and the Construction of Social Reality*, edited by Toni Morrison, 323–63. London: Chatto and Windus.

Lukes, Steven. 1974. *Power: A Radical View*. London: Macmillan.

Lurie, Rachel. 1992. "Translating Issues into Action: Introduction." In *Women, AIDS, and Activism*, edited by ACT UP/New York Women and AIDS Book Group, 211–14. Boston: South End Press.

MacKinnon, Catherine. 1989. *Toward a Feminist Theory of the State*. Cambridge: Harvard University Press.

Maher, Lisa. 1997. *Sexed Work: Gender, Race, and Resistance in a Brooklyn Drug Market*. Oxford: Oxford University Press.

———. 1992. "Reconstructing the Female Criminal: Women and Crack Cocaine." *Southern California Review of Law and Women's Studies* 2, no. 1: 131–54.

Maher, Lisa, and Richard Curtis. 1992. "Women on the Edge of Crime: Crack Cocaine and the Changing Contexts of Street-Level Sex Work in New York City." *Crime, Law and Social Change* 18 (Fall): 222–58.

Maldonado, Lionel A. 1995. "Symposium on West and Fenstermaker's 'Doing Difference.'" *Gender and Society* 9, no. 4 (August): 491–94.

Mauer, Marc, and Tracy Huling. 1995. "Young Black Americans and the Criminal Justice System: Five Years Later: A Report." Washington, D.C.: Sentencing Project.

McBride, David. 1990. *From TB To AIDS: Epidemics among Urban Blacks since 1900*. Albany: State of University of New York Press.

McClaurin, Irma. 2001. *Black Feminist Anthropology: Theory, Politics, Praxis, and Poetics*. New Brunswick, N.J.: Rutgers University Press.

McClintock, Anne. 1993. "Sex Workers and Sex Work: Introduction." *Social Text* 11, no. 4 (Winter): 1–10.

———. 1992. "Screwing the System: Sex Work, Race, and the Law." *Boundary 2*, no. 19 (Summer): 70–95.

McCourt, Kathleen. 1977. *Working Class Women and Grassroots Politics*. Bloomington: Indiana University Press.

Miller, Eleanor. 1986. *Street Woman*. Philadelphia: Temple University Press.

Miller, Jody. 1995. "Gender and Power on the Streets: Street Prostitutes in the Era of Crack Cocaine." *Journal of Contemporary Ethnography* 23 (January): 427–52.

———. 1993. "Your Life Is on the Line Every Night You're on the Streets: Victimization and Resistance among Street Prostitutes." *Humanity and Society* 17, no. 3 (November): 181–96.

Minister, Kristina. 1991. "A Feminist Frame for the Oral History Interview." In *Women's Words: The Feminist Practice of Oral History*, edited by Sherna B. Gluck and Daphne Patai, 27–41. New York: Routledge.

Moraga, Cherrie, and Gloria Anzandula, eds. 1981. *This Bridge Called My Back; Writings By Radical Women of Color*. New York: Kitchen Table Press.

Morgen, Sandra, and Ann Bookman. 1988. "Rethinking Women and Politics: An Introductory Essay." In *Women and the Politics of Empowerment*, edited by Ann Bookman and Sandra Morgen, 3–29. Philadelphia: Temple University Press.

Mumford, K. 1997. *Interzones: Black/White Sex Districts in Chicago and New York in the Early-Twentieth Century*. New York: Columbia University Press.

Murphy, Sheliga, and Marsha Rosenbaum. 1992. "Women Who Use Cocaine Too Much: Smoking Crack versus Snorting Cocaine. *Journal of Psychoactive Drugs* 24, no. 3: 381–88.

———. 1987. "Editors' Introduction: Special Issue: Women and Substance Abuse." *Journal of Psychoactive Drugs* 19, no. 1: 125–28.

Nagle, Jill, ed. 1997. *Whores and Other Feminists*. New York: Routledge.

Naples, Nancy A. 2003. *Feminism and Method: Ethnography, Discourse Analysis, and Activist Research*. New York: Routledge.

———. 1998. "Women's Community Activism: Exploring the Dynamics of Politicization and Diversity." In *Community Activism and Feminist Politics: Organizing across Race, Class, and Gender*, edited by Nancy Naples, 327–49. New York: Routledge.

———. 1992. "Activist Mothering: Cross-Generational Continuity in the Community Work of Women from Low-Income Urban Neighborhoods." *Gender & Society* 6, no. 3: 441–63.

———. 1991a. "Contradictions in the Gender Subtext of the War on Poverty: The Community Work and Resistance of the Women from Low-Income Communities. *Social Problems* 38, no. 3 (August): 316–32.

———. 1991b. " 'Just What Needed to Be Done': The Political Practice of Women Community Workers in Low-Income Neighborhoods." *Gender and Society* 5, no. 4: 478–94.

Nelson, Barbara. 1989. "Women and Knowledge in Political Science: Texts, Histories, and Epistemologies." *Women and Politics* 9, no. 2: 45–67.

Nielsen, L. A. 1984. "Sexual Abuse and Chemical Dependency: Assessing the Risk for Women Alcoholics and Adult Children." *Focus on Family* 7, no. 6: 6–10.

Nyamatha, Adeline, Crystal Benett, Barbara Leake, Charles Lewis, and Jacquelyn Flaskerud. 1993. "AIDS-Related Knowledge, Perceptions, and Behaviors among Impoverished Minority Women." *American Journal of Public Health* 83 (June): 65–71.

O'Leary, Ann, and Patricia Martins. "Structural Factors affecting Women's HIV Risk: A Life Course Example." *AIDS* 14, suppl. 1: 568–72.

Olsen, Tillie. 1979. *Silences*. New York: Delacorte Press/Seymour Lawrence.

Ouellet, Lawrence, Wayne Weibel, Antonio Jimenez, and Wendell Johnson. 1993. "Crack Cocaine and the Transformation of Prostitution in Three Chicago Neighborhoods." In *Crack Pipe as Pimp*, edited by Mitchell S. Ratner, 69–96. New York: Lexington Books.

Paltrow, Lynn. 1990. "When Becoming Pregnant Is a Crime." *Criminal Justice Ethics* 4 (Winter): 41–7.

Passerini, Luisa. 1987. "Women's Personal Narratives: Myths, Experiences, and Emotions." In *Fascism in Popular Memory: The Cultural Experience of the Turin Working Class*. London: Cambridge University Press.

Pardo, Mary. 1998. "Mexican American Women in Eastside Los Angeles." In *Community Activism and Feminist Politics: Organizing across Race, Class, and Gender*, edited by Nancy Naples, 275–300. New York: Routledge.

Park, Sun-Hee Lisa. 1998. "Navigating the Anti-immigrant Wave: The Korean Women's Hotline and the Politics of Community." In *Community Activism and Feminist Politics: Organizing across Race, Class, and Gender*, edited by Nancy Naples, 175–95. New York: Routledge.

Patai, Daphne. 1991. "Us Academics and Third World Women: Is Ethical Research Possible?" In *Women's Words: The Feminist Practice of Oral History*, edited by Sherna B. Gluck and Daphne Patai, 137–53. New York: Routledge.

Patton, Cindy. 1994. *Last Served? Gendering the HIV Pandemic*. London: Taylor and Francis.

Perrow, Charles, Mauro F. Gullien. 1990. *The AIDS Disaster: The Failure of Organizations in New York and the Nation*. New Haven: Yale University.

Personal Narratives Group, The, eds. 1991. *Interpreting Women's Lives: Feminist Theory and Personal Narratives*. Bloomington: Indiana University Press.

Pettigrew, Leon E. 1997. *Workin' It: Women Living through Drugs and Crime*. Philadelphia: Temple University Press, 1997.

Pfuhl, Edwin, and Stuart Henry. 1993. *The Deviance Process*. New York: Aldine De Gruyter.

Pheterson, Gail. 1996. *The Prostitution Prism*. Amsterdam: Amsterdam University Press.

———, ed. 1989. *A Vindication of the Rights of Whores*. Seattle: Seal Press.

Phillips, Pat. 1997. "No Plateau for HIV/AIDS Epidemic in U.S. Women." *Journal of the American Medical Association* 277, no. 22: 1747–49.

Pivnick, Anitra, Audrey Jacobsen, Kathleen Eric, Lynda Doll, and Ernest Drucker. 1994. "AIDS, HIV Infection, and Illicit Drug Use within Inner-City Families and Social Networks." *American Journal of Public Health* 84, no. 2: 271–74.

Plummer, Kenneth. 1975. *Sexual Stigma: An Interactionist Account*. London: Routledge.

Preble, Elizabeth, and Galia D. Siegel. 1996. "Dilemmas for Women in the Second Decade." In *Women's Experiences with HIV/AIDS: An International Perspective*, edited by Lynellyn Long and E. Maxine Ankrah, 297–310. New York: Columbia University Press.

Purnell, Rogaire. 1996. "Child Sexual Abuse, Alcohol and Drug (Mis)Use, and Human Immunodeficiency Virus (HIV) Vulnerability among African-American Women: An Exploratory Study. Ph.D. dissertation. University of Michigan.

Quam, M. 1990. "The Sick Role, Stigma, and Pollution: The Case of AIDS." In *Culture and AIDS*, edited by D. Feldman. New York: Praeger.

Queen, Carol. 1997. "Sex Radical Politics, Sex-Positive Feminist Thought and Whore Stigma," In *Whores and Other Feminists*, edited by Jill Nagle, 125–35. New York: Routledge.

Randall, Vicky. 1987. *Women and Politics: An International Perspective*. London: Macmillan Education.

Rapping, Elayne. 1996. *The Culture of Recovery: Making Sense of the Self-Help Movement in Women's Lives*. Boston: Beacon Press.

Ratner, Mitchell S., ed. 1993. *Crack Pipe as Pimp*. New York: Lexington Books.

Reeves, Jimmie L., and Richard Campbell. 1994. *Cracked Coverage: Television News, the Anti-Cocaine Crusade, and the Reagan Legacy*. Durham, N.C.: Duke University Press.

Rich, Adrienne. 1979. *On Lies, Secrets, and Silence: Selected Prose, 1966–1978*. New York: Norton.

Richardson, Laurel. 1990. *Writing Strategies: Reaching Diverse Audiences*. Newberry Park, Calif.: Sage Publications.

Richie, Beth E. 1996. *Compelled to Crime: The Gender Entrapment of Battered Black Women*. New York: Routledge.

Riley, Denise. 1988. *"Am I That Name?": Feminism and the Category of "Woman" in History*. Minneapolis: University of Minnesota Press.

Risseman, Catherine Kohler. 1987. "When Gender Is Not Enough: Women Interviewing Women." *Gender and Society* 1, no. 3: 172–207.

Roberts, Dorothy. 1991. "Punishing Drug Addicts Who Have Babies: Women of Color, Equality, and the Right of Privacy." *Harvard Law Review* 104, no. 9: 1419–34.

Rohsenow, D. J., R. Corbett, and D. Devine. 1988. "Molested as Children: A Hidden Contribution to Substance Abuse." *Journal of Substance Abuse Treatment* 5: 13–18.

Rosen, R. 1982. *The Lost Sisterhood: Prostitution in America, 1900–1918*. Baltimore: Johns Hopkins University Press.

Rosenberg, Phillip. 1995. "Scope of AIDS Epidemic in the United States." *Science* 270, no. 3: 1372–75.

Rosenstone, Steve, and John Mark Hansen. 1993. *Mobilization, Participation, and Democracy in America*. New York: Macmillan Publishing Company.

Sachs, Karen Brodkin. 1988. "Gender and Grassroots Leadership." In *Women and The Politics of Empowerment*, edited by Ann Bookman and Sandra Morgen, 77–94. Philadelphia: Temple University Press.

Sacks, Valerie. 1996. "Women and AIDS: An Analysis of Media Misrepresentations." *Social Science and Medicine* 42, no. 1: 59–73.

Sargent, Robert, James L. Sorensen, Brian Greenberg, Gwen Evans, Alfonso P. Acampora. 1999. "Residential Detoxification for Substance Abusers with HIV/AIDS: Walden House Detoxification Program." *Journal of Substance Abuse Treatment* 16 (January): 87–95.

Schneider, Beth E., and Nancy Stoller, eds. 1995. *Women Resisting AIDS: Feminist Strategies of Empowerment*. Philadelphia: Temple University Press.

———. 1995. "Introduction: Feminist Strategies of Empowerment." In *Women Resisting AIDS: Feminist Strategies of Empowerment*, edited by Beth E. Schneider and Nancy Stoller, 1–20. Philadelphia: Temple University Press.

Schlozman, Kay Lehman, Nancy Burns, and Sidney Verba. 1994. "Gender and Pathways to Participation: The Role of Resources." *Journal of Politics* 56, no. 4: 963–90.

Schur, Edwin. 1983. *Labeling Women Deviant: Gender, Stigma, and Social Control*. Philadelphia: Temple University Press.

———. 1980. *The Politics of Deviance*. Englewood Cliffs, N.J.: Prentice-Hall.

Shaw, Nancy Stoller. 1988. "Preventing AIDS among Women: The Role of Community Organizing." *Socialist Review* 100 (Fall): 76–92.

Shayne, V. T., and B. J. Kaplan. 1991. "Double Victims: Poor Women with AIDS." *Women's Health* 17, no. 10: 21–27.

Sherr, Lorraine, Catherine Hawkins, and Lydia Bennett, eds. 1996. *AIDS as a Gender Issue: Psychosocial Perspectives*. London: Taylor and Francis.

Silliman, Jael, Anannya Bhattachrajee, and Angela Davis, eds. 2002. *Policing the National Body: Race, Gender, and Criminalization*. Cambridge, Mass.: South End Press.

Smith, Barbara, ed. 1983. *Home Girls: A Black Feminist Anthology*. New York: Kitchen Table Press.

Smith, Dorothy E. 1987. *The Everyday World as Problematic: A Feminist Sociology*. Boston: Northeastern University Press.

Sosnowitz, Barbara. G. 1995. "AIDS Prevention, Minority Women, and Gender Assertiveness." In *Women Resisting AIDS: Feminist Strategies of Empowerment*, edited by Beth Schneider and Nancy Stoller, 139–61. Philadelphia: Temple University Press.

Sotelo-Hondagneu, Pierrette. 1998. "Latina Immigrant Women and Paid Domestic Work: Upgrading the Occupation." In *Community Activism and Feminist Politics: Organizing across Race, Class and Gender*, edited by Nancy Naples, 199–211. New York: Routledge.

Speed-Castillo, Lillian. 1995. *Latina: Voices from the Borderlands*. New York: Simon and Schuster.

Spillers, Hortense. 1984. "Interstices: A Small Drama of Words." In *Pleasure and Danger*, edited by Carole Vance, 73–100. Boston: Routledge and Kegan Paul.

Spivak, Gayatri Chakravorty. 1998. *In Other Worlds: Essays in Cultural Politics*. New York: Routledge.

Spradley. J. P. 1979. *The Ethnographic Interview*. New York: Holt, Rinehart and Winston.

Stacey, Judith. 1991. "Can There Be a Feminist Ethnography?" In *Women's Words: The Feminist Practice of Oral History*, edited by Sherna B. Gluck and Daphne Patai, 111–19. New York: Routledge.

Stafford, Mark C., and Richard Scott. 1986. "Stigma, Deviance, and Social Control: Some Conceptual Issues." In *The Dilemma of Difference: A Multidisciplinary*

View of Stigma, edited by Stephen Ainlay, Gaylene Becker, and Lerita Coleman, 78–90. New York: Plenum Press.

Stern, Susan Parkison. 1998. "Conversation, Research, and Struggles over Schooling in an African American Community." In *Community Activism and Feminist Politics: Organizing across Race, Class and Gender*, edited by Nancy Naples, 107–27. New York: Routledge.

Strauss, Anslem, and Juliet Corbin. 1997. *Grounded Theory in Practice*. Thousand Oaks, Calif.: Sage Publications.

Stoller, Nancy E. 1998. *Lessons from the Damned: Queers, Whores, and Junkies Respond to AIDS*. New York: Routledge.

———. 1995. "Lesbian Involvement in the AIDS Epidemic: Changing Roles and Generational Differences." In *Women Resisting AIDS: Feminist Strategies of Empowerment*, edited by Beth E. Schneider and Nancy Stoller, 270–85. Philadelphia: Temple University Press.

Sudbury, Julia. 2001. "(Re)constructing Multiracial Blackness: Women's Activism, Difference, and Collective Identity in Britain." *Ethnic and Racial Studies* 24, no. 1: 29–49.

Sumpter, Bambi. 1992. "We Have a Job to Do." In *Women, AIDS, and Activism*. ACT UP/New York Women and AIDS Book Group, 223–25. Boston: South End Press.

Susser, Ida. 1988. "Working-Class Women, Social Protest, and Changing Ideologies." In *Women and The Politics of Empowerment*, edited by Ann Bookman and Sandra Morgen, 257–71. Philadelphia: Temple University Press.

Takagi, Dana Y. 1995. "Symposium on West and Fenstermaker's 'Doing Difference.'" *Gender and Society* 9, no. 5 (August): 496–97.

Taylor, Verta, and Leila J. Rupp. 1998. "Women's Culture and Lesbian Feminist Activism: A Reconsideration of Cultural Feminism." In *Community Activism and Feminist Politics: Organizing across Race, Class, and Gender*, edited by Nancy Naples, 57–79. New York: Routledge.

Thorne, Barrie. 1995. "Symposium on West and Fenstermaker's 'Doing Difference.'" *Gender and Society* 9 no. 5 (August): 497–99.

Titmus, Ronald. 1974. *Social Policy Analysis: An Introduction*. New York: Pantheon Books.

Tonry, Michael, and Joan Petersilia, eds. 2000. *Prisons: Crime and Justice*. Chicago: University of Chicago Press.

Travers, Michele, and Lydia Bennett. 1996. "AIDS, Women, and Power." In *AIDS as a Gender Issue: Psychosocial Perspectives*, edited by Lorraine Sherr, Catherine Hankins, and Lydia Bennett, 64–77. London: Taylor and Francis.

Troung, Than Dam. 1990. *Sex, Money, and Morality: The Political Economy of Prostitution and Tourism in Southeast Asia*. London: Zed Books.

Twine, Frances Winddance, and Johnathan Warren. 2000. *Racing Research, Researching Race: Methodological Dilemmas in Critical Race Studies*. New York: New York University Press.

Valdiserri, Ronald. 2002. "HIV/AIDS Stigma: An Impediment to Public Health." *American Journal of Public Health* 92, no. 3 (March): 341–42.

Wadsworth, R., A. M. Spamento, and B. M. Halbrook. 1995. "The Role of Sexual Trauma in the Treatment of Chemically Dependent Women: Addressing the Relapse Issue. *Journal of Counseling and Development* 73: 401–06.

Wagner, D. 1990. *The Quest for a Radical Profession: Social Service Careers and Political Ideology*. Lanham, Md.: University Press of America.

Walker, Alice. 1983. *In Search of Our Mothers' Gardens*. New York: Harcourt Brace Jovanovich.

Wallace, Michele. 1992. "*Boyz N the Hood and Jungle Fever*." In *Black Popular Culture*, edited by Gina Dent, 123–30. Seattle: Bay Press.

———. 1990. *Invisibility Blues: From Pop to Theory*. New York: Verso.

Warren, Carol A. B. 1988. *Gender Issues in Field Research*. Newbury Park, Calif.: Sage Publications.

Weber, Lynn. 1995. "Symposium on West and Fenstermaker's 'Doing Difference.'" *Gender and Society* 9, no. 5 (August): 491–94.

Weitz, Rose. 1995. "Coping with AIDS." In *Down To Earth Sociology*, edited by James M. Henslin. New York: Free Press.

West, Candace, and Sarah Fenstermaker. 1995a. "Doing Difference." *Gender and Society* 9, no. 5 (August): 8–37.

———. 1995b. "Symposium on West and Fenstermaker's 'Doing Difference'—Reply." *Gender and Society* 9, no. 5 (August): 491–94.

———. 1993. "Power, Inequality, and the Accomplishment of Gender: An Ethnomethodological View." In *Theory on Gender: Feminism on Theory*, edited by Paula England. Hawthrone: Aldine de Gruyter.

West, Guida, and Rhoda Lois Blumberg. 1990. "Reconstructing Social Protest from a Feminist Perspective." In *Women and Social Protest*, edited by Guida West and Rhoda Lois Blumberg, 3–35. New York: Oxford University Press.

White, Lucie. 1990. *The Comforts of Home: Prostitution in Colonial Nairobi*. Chicago: University of Chicago Press.

Williams, Patricia. 1991. *The Alchemy of Race and Rights: Diary of a Law Professor*. Cambridge: Harvard University Press.

Winant, Howard. 1995. "Symposium on West and Fenstermaker's 'Doing Difference.'" *Gender and Society* 9, no. 5 (August): 493–96.

Wittner, Judith. 1998. "Reconceptualizing Agency in Domestic Violence Court." In *Community Activism and Feminist Politics: Organizing across Race, Class, and Gender*, edited by Nancy Naples, 81–104. New York: Routledge.

Wolfe, Maxine. 1992. "AIDS and Politics: Transformation of Our Movement." In *Women, AIDS, and Activism*, edited by ACT UP/New York Women and AIDS Book Group, 233–37. Boston: South End Press.

Worth, Dooley. 1990. "Minority Women and AIDS: Culture, Race, and Gender." *In Culture and AIDS*, edited by Douglas A. Feldman, 111–136. New York: Praeger.

Young, Iris Marion. 1994. "Punishment, Treatment, Empowerment: Three Approaches to Policy for Pregnant Addicts." *Feminist Studies* 20, no. 1: 33–57.

Zachery-Jordan, Julia S. 2001. "Black Womanhood and Social Welfare Policy: The Influence of Her Image on Policy Making." *Sage Race Relations Abstracts* 26, no. 3: 5–24.

Zerai, Assata, and Rae Banks. 2002. *Dehumanizing Discourse, Anti-Drug Law and Policy in America: "A Crack Mother's Nightmare."* Burlington, Vt.: Aldershot.

Zinn, Maxine Baca, and Bonnie Thornton Dill, eds. 1994. *Women of Color in U.S. Society*. Philadelphia: Temple University Press.

Index

academia: sex work research stigmatized in, 77–79
Ackelsberg, Martha, 185, 187
ACLU (American Civil Liberties Union), 157
Acquired Immunodeficiency Syndrome. *See* AIDS; HIV/AIDS
activists and activism: activities and roles of, 12–13, 174–80; advocacy compared with, 152; appearances by, 117; bio-sketches of, 50–58; on breast cancer and HIV/AIDS, compared, 106–7; challenges of, 151; definitions of political, 83–84; as experiential, 181–82; obstacles to, 139–42; use of term, 18, 144. *See also* Cherise (respondent); Daria (respondent); Kitt (respondent); Shenna (respondent)
ACT-UP, 32, 124
advocates and advocacy: activism compared with, 152; activities and roles of, 12, 116–17; beginnings of, 105, 154–56; bio-sketches of, 38–50; blended and overlapping roles of, 151–54; challenges of, 151, 160; as experiential, 181–82; issues in, 156–58; non-organizational or agency, 163–69; as paid and unpaid, 153–54, 160–63; training for, 116–18, 167–68. *See also* Billy Jean (respondent); Charlene (respondent); Constance (respondent); Julianna (respondent); Nicole (respondent); Valerie (respondent)
African American community: church as moral authority in, 170, 199–200n.34; epidemics as perceived by, 206n.5; lesbians and gays in, 51, 175; public institutions and, 206n.4; women's activism in, 9–10
African American women: AIDS crisis for, 7; as center of narratives, 182–84; community activism of, 9–10; constructing identity of, 34–35, 199–200n.34; as first wave of HIV-positive women, 184; popular representations of, 77, 202n.16. *See also* respondents

agencies and organizations: advocacy via, 160–63; interactions among, 164; list of, 193–94; on sex workers' rights, 35; structural problems in, 165–66. *See also* churches; leadership and leadership skills; *specific agencies and organizations*
AIDS (Acquired Immunodeficiency Syndrome): metaphors for, 28. *See also* HIV/AIDS
AIDS Awareness Workshop, 71–72, 155–56
AIDS Quilt project, 142, 178
Ain't Nobody's Business, 176
alcohol abuse: recovery programs on, 112; respondents on, 39, 43, 52, 56, 60, 62, 200n.2. *See also* substance abuse treatment
Alonzo, Angelo, 25, 28
American Civil Liberties Union (ACLU), 157
Anderson, Kathryn, 81, 82, 84
Anna (respondent): bio-sketch of, 62; on black women, 184; as child with adult responsibilities, 201n.17; on diagnosis, 95; as helper, 173–74; on sexual abuse, 111; on stigma, 121; on substance abuse treatment, 107
arts: activism via, 174, 178–79; advocacy via, 169; fund-raising via, 178; social issues addressed in, 207n.20
Austin, Regina, 25–26

Bambara, Toni Cade, 119
Barbarella (film), 138
Battle, Shelia, 102, 204n.19
Beale, Frances, 197n.17
"being a woman with HIV" phrase, 134, 136, 205n.11
Bell, Shannon, 34
Billy Jean (respondent): advocacy and, 117; bio-sketch of, 48–50; on children and marriage, 120; on diagnosis, 97–98; difficulties of, 139–40, 188; on HIV status, 100–101, 104; on male partner, 120, 133; on politics, 148
Black Power movement, 197n.17
blended and overlapping roles: advocacy in, 151–54; concept of, 12–13, 83–84,

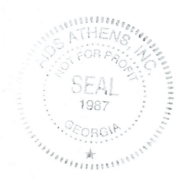